The Second Mile

40-Days+ of Fitness and Faith

Sheila and Peter Roesler

Friends for Better Health's Step by Step Guide to Wellness

Do your part and let our heavenly Father do the supernatural

Facts, Challenges, Recipes, Scriptural Helps, Check Lists,

and Room for Personal Prayers and Challenges

"I will praise thee, for I am fearfully, and wonderfully made…" (Ps. 139:14).

"I beseech you therefore, brethren, by the mercies of God,
that ye present your bodies a living sacrifice, holy, acceptable unto God,
which is your reasonable service." (Rom. 12:1).

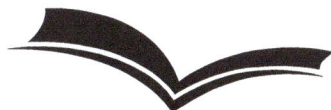

TEACH Services, Inc.
PUBLISHING
www.TEACHServices.com ● (800) 367-1844

_____

Copyright © 2020 Peter and Sheila Roesler

Copyright © 2020 TEACH Services, Inc.

ISBN-13: 978-1-4796-1256-7 (Paperback)

ISBN-13: 978-1-4796-1257-4 (ePub)

Library of Congress Control Number: 2020914205

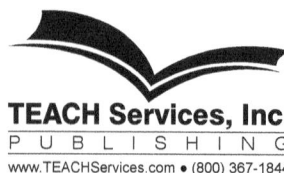

TEACH Services, Inc.
PUBLISHING
www.TEACHServices.com ● (800) 367-1844

Table of Contents

Foreword

You can start the program anytime. It is highly recommended to continue for the entire forty days. Prayer and developing a close relationship with our Heavenly Father will ensure success to better health as you FOLLOW HIS STEPS.

Our aim is to motivate your choice to follow a healthier lifestyle for yourself. We can only inform and encourage…we cannot make you do anything. However, if you would like to be motivated, just ask our Father in heaven for the desire. It is as simple as that.

We created the book in a simple format so that day by day you can incorporate special activities into your life. The change takes time. There must be balance in the lifestyle. The need for symmetrical balance is why the program includes mental, physical, and spiritual (moral) information and activities.

Sheila Roesler (formally known as Sheila Maynard), is a native of Barbados, West Indies. At the age of thirteen, God inspired her to become a medical missionary doctor. Her journey began when she came to the United States over forty-nine years ago. Educated in New York City, she then received her BA from Brandeis University and her master's in education, with an emphasis in urban youth development, from National University. She is a "Who's Who in American Teachers" award winner. She taught high school math and science, and was the former owner of a Kumon Math franchise. She was a research associate at Harvard School of Public Health in the nutrition and epidemiology departments.

Sheila has been teaching God's preventive health principles in the settings of dynamic health empowerment parties, vegan cooking classes, seminars, workshops, and private consultations in homes, schools, churches, and organizations across the United States and abroad for over twenty-five years.

Peter Roesler was born in Washington state but grew up in northern California. He received his BA and master's in industrial education from Pacific Union College. He spent many missionary years in the islands of Micronesia as a teacher and builder. He was a professor and high school teacher in the United States as well.

Peter and Sheila have been married five years and together they are ministering in the world field and on the "Faith Farm." Everything they do is by faith.

They both have received training as medical missionaries and are now educating the public on a local television show, at churches, and in homes on "Living God's Preventive Hygienic Health Principles."

All is done "In His Majesty's Service."

Introduction

"Let us hear the conclusion of the whole matter: **Fear God and keep His commandments:** for this is the whole duty of man. For God shall bring every work into judgement with every secret thing, whether it be good, or whether it be evil" (Eccles. 12:13, 14, bold added for emphasis).

What is your reward? "Blessed are they that do his commandments, that they may have right to the tree of life, and may enter in through the gates into the city" (Rev. 22:14).

What are His commandments? They are physical, mental, and moral. When they are violated, the sickness, disease, violence, and all ills creep into our bodies and homes. 2 Corinthians 4:6 says, "For God, who commanded the light to shine out of darkness, (in the beginning), hath shined in our hearts, to give the light of the knowledge of the glory of God in the face (image) of Jesus Christ (Our Savior and Redeemer)" (parenthetical words added for clarity).

Our aim in the Second Mile 40-Days+ Wellness Program, is to share some of the knowledge of the glory of God. He says in 1 Corinthians 10:31, "Whether therefore ye eat, or drink, or whatsoever ye do, do all to the glory of God."

You invested in this program because you are investing in your life here on earth and for the future kingdom. The road is not smooth; there are many bumps and obstacles along the way. One of the biggest obstacles is yourself. Yes, you have been holding yourself back from a beautiful healthy life. Now you have chosen to change your lifestyle. You have chosen to surrender all unhealthy habits to your Savior. Yes, you must give them up to Him. There are just a few simple things to do.

First, confess them to yourself and to God. He already knows, but He has been patiently waiting for you to admit that you like to eat a lot of the wrong things, drink unhealthy beverages, even look at things that corrupt and pollute your mind. We are going to pay closer attention to those five gates that allow the enemy of our souls to enter. These consist of the eye gate, the ear gate, the nose gate, the mouth gate, and the touch gate. These are your senses. Ask the Father who created you to forgive you for not respecting His creation: you.

Secondly, be repentant. Take time to think and pray about how much sickness and stress you have allowed to enter into your body, mind, and soul.

Thirdly, pray and ask the Father to show you where you have gone off course. Ask Him to help you turn from those habits which prevent Him from fulfilling His perfect and healthy plan for you. The promise He give in Deuteronomy 28:1, 2 applies to you, too. "And it shall come to pass, if thou shalt hearken diligently unto the voice of the Lord (Yah) thy God (Elohiym), to observe and do all His commandments which I (Moses) command thee this day, that the Lord thy God will set thee on high above all nations of the earth: And all these blessings shalt come on thee, and overtake thee, if thou shalt hearken unto the voice of the Lord thy God."

You will have all the help you need. First, God will give you a new heart if you ask. Read Psalm 51 a few times. Then, as God delights to do, He will GIVE. "And I will give them one heart, and I will put a new spirit within you; and I will take the stony heart out of their flesh, and will give them an heart of flesh: That they may walk in my statutes, and keep mine ordinances, and do them: and they shall be my people, and I will be their God" (Ezek. 11:19, 20).

After this, surrender so our Father can call you His own. You might have done this before or thought you were already walking in His way, but if you have been "self-murdering" yourself, you have not being making God your Father. Remember, and this is hard to say, but the Father of lies was the first murderer and we do not want to be his children (John 8:44).

You do know that "with God all things are possible" (Mark 10:27). Our Savior and Redeemer has already won the victory for us. Remember how you rode the back of an older sibling or parent when you were little, and he or she would win the race for you? The joy of winning was yours even though you did not put your feet on the ground during the race. Well, the joy of being victorious in this race is yours too, even though you do not have to fast forty days or suffer death on the cross. Praise God for all He has done for us and will do for us. Your heart should be overwhelmed here. Just think of it: Jesus went without food or drink for forty days, which is almost six weeks. He is not requiring that of us today, but I know we can eat our way to health in less than six weeks. Yeshua (His Hebrew name), is not requiring that of us today. During this time, you will (I know you will) receive significant benefits from following His program.

Our wellness program lasts for 40 days. It is a lifestyle change that will restore, revitalize, and rebuild your body. It will involve new physical practices, new mental exercises, and hopefully a totally new moral outlook on life that will affect you, and those around you.

HOLD ON. Stay with us and we can begin this journey together.

It starts with prayer. We will pray about **everything**. This simply means that we will talk to God about **everything**—Yes, **everything**.

First, we must make sure we know where He is and who we are talking to. We must direct our prayers to God, the Father in heaven. Remember that "God was in Christ, reconciling the world unto himself, not imputing (charging) their trespasses (sins) unto them; and hath committed unto us the word of reconciliation" (2 Cor. 5:19). So, "Seeing then that we have a great high priest, that is passed into the heavens, Jesus the Son of God, let us hold fast our profession. For we have not an high priest that cannot be touched with the feeling of our infirmities; but was in all points tempted like as we are, yet without sin" (Heb. 4:14, 15). He was tempted with the lust of the eyes (appetite), the lust of the flesh (lust or coveting) and the pride of life (wanting the best and to be first) (see Matt. 4).

The greatest test seems to be appetite. The enemy of our soul seems to think that it would be the easiest method since it worked so well with Adam and Eve (Gen. 3:1). However, our great High Priest and Savior did not take the bait. He won the victory over appetite for us: "…yet learned he obedience by the things which he suffered" (Heb. 5:8). "Let us therefore come boldly unto the throne of grace, that we may obtain mercy, and find grace to help in time of need" (Heb. 4:16).

We are coming boldly to offer our prayers. Ask the Almighty Father to help you each day with the program. Just take one day at a time.

As you incorporate these health principles into your daily routine, start prayerfully. Part of the program is to incorporate the habit of going the second mile (see Matt. 5:41) for a friend, stranger, or your neighbor. Remember that your closest neighbor is the one who lives with you.

It is outlined as follows:

Forgive Others

Offer Praise and Thanksgiving

Lend a Helping Hand

Love Life

Obey Willingly

Wear Healthy Clothes

Healthy Foods

Intimacy with God

Sweet Sleep

Soft Water

Temperance Always

Exercise Daily

Pure, Fresh Air

Sunlight

A **SECOND MILE ACT** should be from the heart. It can be a chore, an errand, something you do for your spouse, children, partner, friends, relatives, or enemies. It could be the giving of money, clothes, time, food, or a smile and a kind word. Make it a matter of prayer to let the Lord lead you.

> **"PRAYER** is the key in the hand of faith to unlock heaven's storehouse, where are treasured the boundless resources of Omnipotence. Without unceasing prayer and diligent watching, we are in danger of growing careless and of deviating from the right path" (White, *Steps to Christ*, p. 94).

> "Let the soul be drawn out and upward, that God may grant us a breath of the heavenly atmosphere. We may keep so near to God that in every unexpected trial our thoughts will turn to Him as naturally as the flower turns to the sun" (White, *Steps to Christ*, p. 99).

> > Keep your wants, your joys, your sorrows, your cares, and your fears before God. You cannot burden Him; you cannot weary Him. He who numbers the hairs of your head is not indifferent to the wants of His children. "The Lord is very pitiful, and of tender mercy." James 5:11. His heart of love is touched by our sorrows and even by our utterances of them. Take to Him everything that perplexes the mind. Nothing is too great for Him to bear, for He holds up worlds, He rules over all the affairs of the universe. Nothing that in any way concerns our peace is too small for Him to notice. There is no chapter in our experience too dark for Him to read; there is no perplexity too difficult for Him to unravel. No calamity can befall the least of His children, no anxiety harass the soul, no joy cheer, no sincere prayer escape the lips, of which our heavenly Father is unobservant, or in which He takes no immediate interest. "He healeth the broken in heart, and bindeth up their wounds." Psalm 147:3. The relations between God and each soul are as distinct and full as though there were not another soul upon the earth to share His watch care, not another soul for whom He gave His beloved Son. (White, *Steps to Christ*, p. 100)

A Sample Prayer to Overcome

Heavenly Father,

Thank You for Your blessings in my life.

I thank You for Your mercy and long-suffering towards me and for the merit of the sacrifice of Jesus Christ, who died for my sins.

Please forgive me for_____ (for example, not drinking water).

Please cover all my sins with the precious blood of Jesus Christ.

I am so sorry I sinned against Him and You.

I confess that I have the desire to _____ (Name the desire. Be specific.).

Please give me the power of Your Holy Spirit to overcome _____ (Name the habit.).

Please increase my faith in the righteousness and grace of Jesus Christ to help me overcome.

Please give me the strength to_____ (for example: drink more water; name the habit you want to change).

In the name of Jesus Christ or Yeshua, Amen.

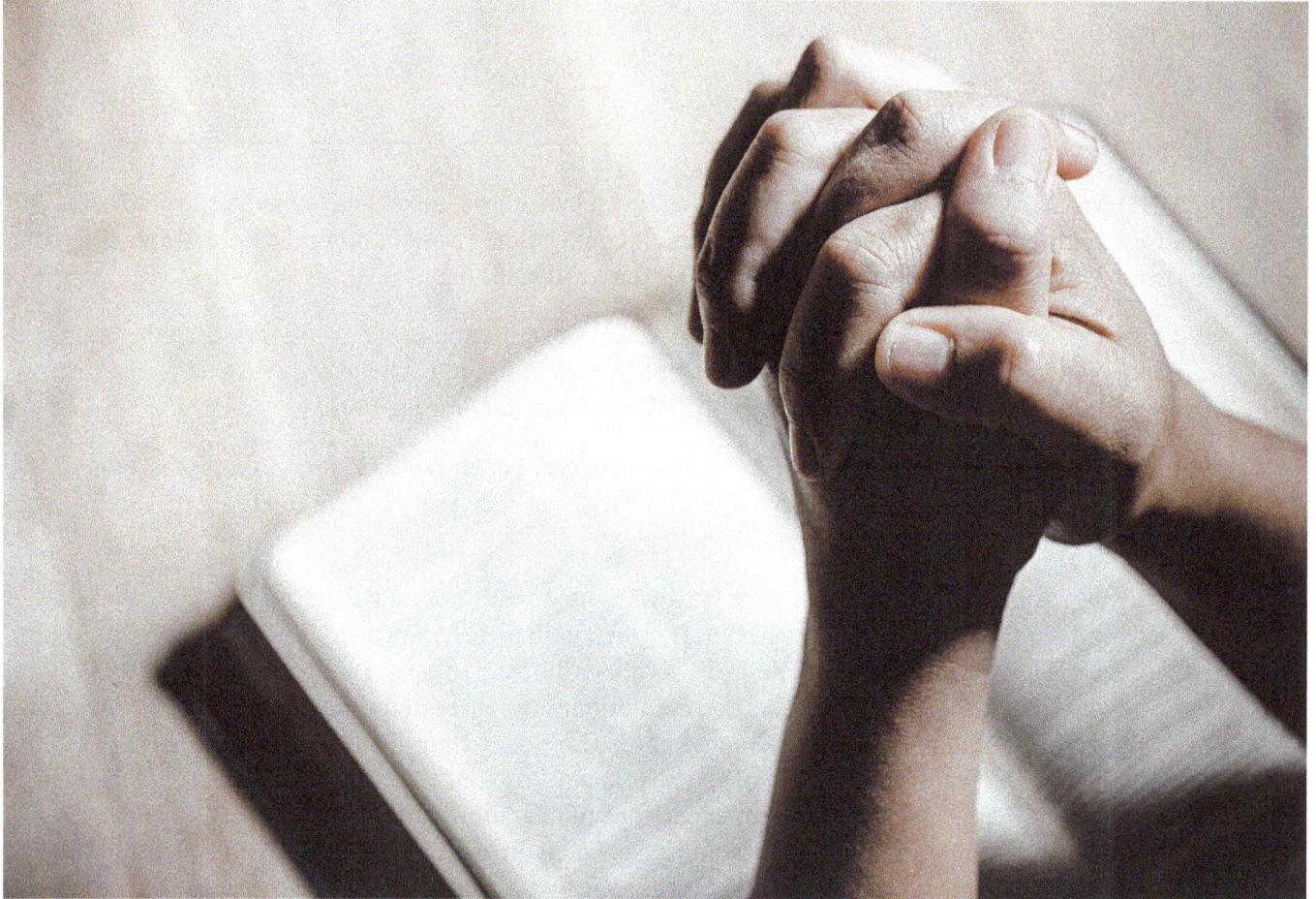

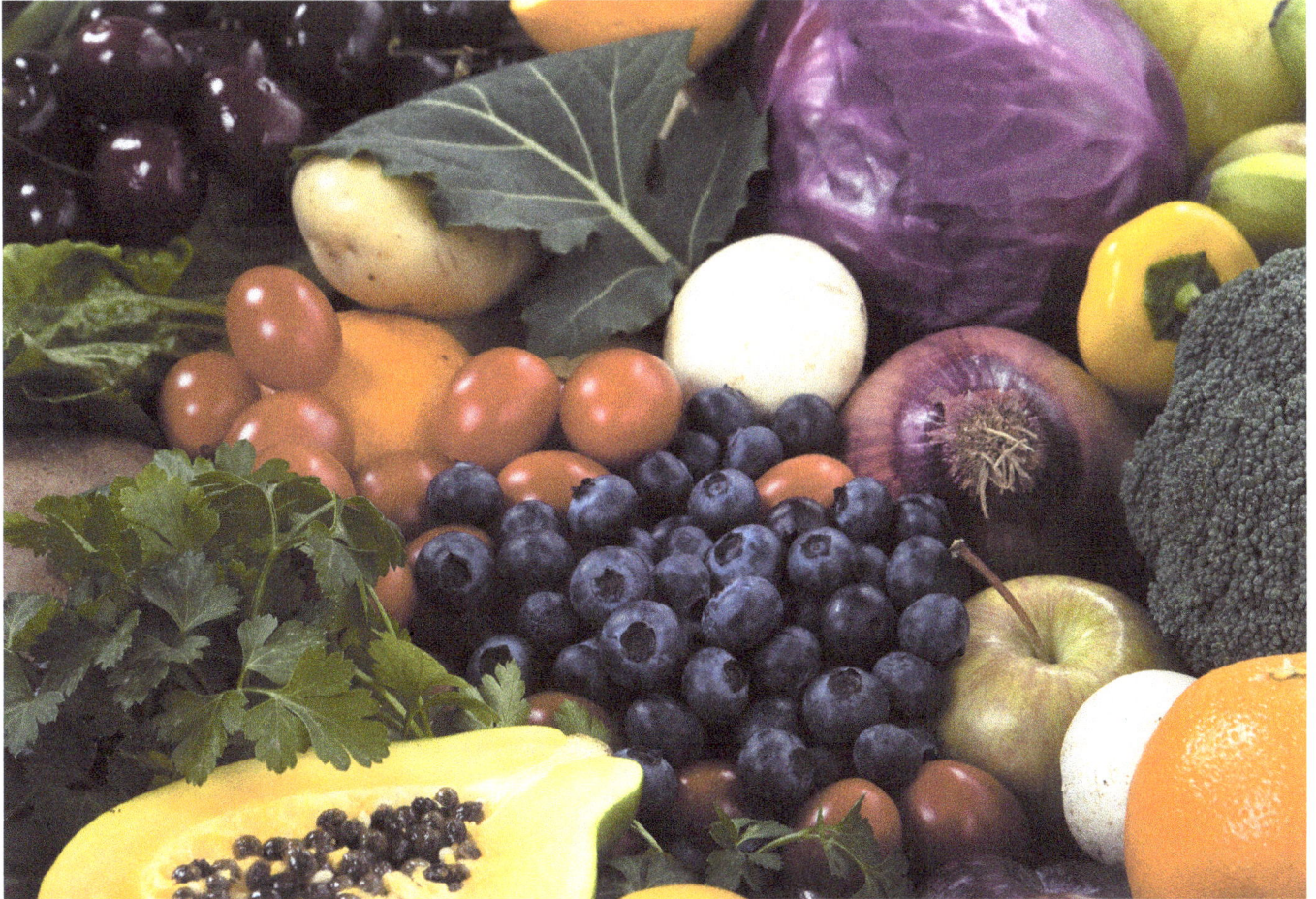

Healthy Foods

"And God said, Behold, I have given you every herb bearing seed, which is upon the face of all the earth, and every tree, in the which is the fruit of a tree yielding seed; to you it shall be for meat" (Gen. 1:29).

The building blocks of the body are contained in the food we eat. Good nutrition is easy to come by if we eat regularly and simply. Food was provided to maintain good health, not to indulge appetite.

FACTS ABOUT HEALTHY FOODS (Ferrell and Cherne 2010)

1. Avoid refined foods or even enriched foods. They are void of most nutrients.

2. As much as possible, use the food in its natural form, such as fruits, vegetables, nuts, seeds, grains, and legumes (beans). These foods fight disease.

3. Fresh fruits and vegetables are preferred. Frozen is the next best option. Canned fruits and vegetables in their natural juices are good alternatives. Eating steamed fruits and vegetables are excellent alternatives for you to get your nutrients if your teeth or gums prevent you from chewing fresh fruits and vegetables.

4. Avoid as much second-hand food as possible (like fish, chicken, and other meats).

5. Cook in stainless steel, corning ware, glass, or iron pans. Do not use aluminum cookware.

6. Avoid protein from animal sources. These provide an excess of fat, cholesterol, and protein; yes, excess protein. They often carry harmful viruses and bacteria, as well as hormones, antibiotics, and other chemical substances.

7. Eat a queen's breakfast, a king's lunch, and a pauper's supper; preferably NO SUPPER.

8. There should be five to six hours between meals, allowing the stomach to have time to digest the food and to rest.

9. The lightest meal should be in the evening, at least three to four hours before bedtime.

10. Do not drink fluids with meals. It slows down the digestive processes. Do not drink within a half hour before eating and wait at least an hour after eating.

11. **Do not eat between meals.** If your blood sugar gets low, have a little juice or fruit.

12. **DO NOT EAT VINEGAR** OR ITS PRODUCTS. Vinegar causes fermentation in the stomach and the food does not digest, but instead decays and putrefies. The blood is therefore not nourished, but becomes filled with impurities, and then the liver and kidney begins to have difficulties.

13. Use lemon or lime juice as a substitute for vinegar.

14. **DO NOT EAT UNNATURAL MARGARINE.** It blocks the entrance of nutrients into the cells.

PHYSICAL AWARENESS

My Current Health Assessment

1. Do you eat any meat or flesh (i.e. chicken, turkey, pork, fish, shrimp, etc.)? Yes/No

2. Do you eat any dairy or eggs (i.e. milk, cheese, yogurt, chocolate, etc.)? Yes/No

3. Do you eat refined white products (i.e. white bread, white rice, white flour items)? Yes/No

4. How many servings do you eat per day of fruit _____ of vegetables _____?

5. Do you use condiments (i.e. ketchup, mustard, mayonnaise, barbeque sauces, salad dressings, pickles, vinegar, etc.)? Yes/No

6. Do you eat fried foods often? Yes/No

7. Do you use margarine or butter? Yes/No

8. Do you eat fresh (made within twenty-four hrs.) bread? Yes/No

9. Do you eat or drink any cocoa, chocolate, or ice cream? Yes/No; How often? _____

10. Which oils do you cook with? _____

11. Do you read the labels of food items you buy from the store? Yes/No

12. Circle any sweeteners you eat (i.e. sugar, honey, Splenda®, Sweet'n Low®, Equal®)

13. Do you eat nuts with each meal? Yes/No

14. Do you eat any canned items (beans, veggies, fruits, veggie meats, etc.)? Yes/No

15. Are you on any special diet? Yes/No

16. Do you eat out or eat carry-out often? Yes/No

17. Do you use salt? Yes/No

18. Does the salt contain iodine? Yes/No

YOUR CHALLENGES ARE:

__to eat more fresh veggies at one meal.

__to eat more fresh fruit at my next meal.

__to avoid regular salt (The body needs salt, but not refined salt.).

__to reduce fried food intake.

__to do a **SECOND MILE ACT** for someone:

__**to claim this promise:** *"If any of you lack wisdom, let him ask of God…and it shall be given him"* (James 1:5).

RECIPES FOR THE DAY:

CORN BUTTER/MARGARINE

2–3 Tbsp. hot water

2 Tbsp. coconut cream/milk or oil

½ tsp. salt

¼ tsp. garlic powder

1 cup freshly cooked corn meal or fresh or frozen corn

BLEND the first 4 ingredients until creamy; add the corn and continue blending until smooth. POUR into container, cover, and chill in refrigerator for one hour.

MAKING THE SALAD and DRESSING TOGETHER

First, add olive oil, salt, and lemon juice to your greens (especially kale and arugula).

MASSAGE the greens. This reduces the amount of greens, so now you will eat more greens when you fill your bowl. ADD the additional ingredients, plus some honey and nuts. (Optional: Add your special salad dressing.)

FRENCH DRESSING

½ cup oil

2 Tbsp. sesame seeds

1½ tsp. paprika

1½ Tbsp. onion powder

¼ to ½ cup lemon juice

2 Tbsp. honey

1 tsp. salt

BLEND until creamy.

MENTAL & MORAL AWARENESS

Together, we will be dealing with the mental and moral awareness aspect of our program. They have a remarkable effect on each other.

The brain is the center, or ruler, of the body. It is the seat of all the nervous forces and of mental action. The nerves coming out from the brain control the body. By the brain nerves, our mental impressions are conveyed to all other nerves of the body like telegraph wires. They control the vital action of every part of the system. All the organs of motion are governed by the communications they receive from the brain. The brain nerves are the only medium through which heaven can communicate with man that affects the entire life physically, mentally and morally. Whatever disturbs the circulation of the electric currents in the nervous system lessens the strength of the vital powers and deadens the sensibilities of the mind.

Prayer is a mental and moral activity so we will cover it during this section throughout the program.

We will follow Christ's steps through the sanctuary as outlined in the Old Testament, and which continues in heaven RIGHT NOW.

WHAT DOES THE BIBLE SAY?

The Sanctuary

- Why did God tell Moses to build a Sanctuary *(Ex. 25:8)*?
- Describe the Sanctuary *(Heb. 9:1–5)*.
- What was inside the ark *(Deut. 10:4, 5)*?
- How were sins forgiven at that time *(Lev. 4:27–30)*?
- What is Jesus doing now *(Dan. 8:14, Heb. 9:24)*?

✓ *DAILY WELLNESS CHECK*

__Did I eat more fruits and vegetables today?

MY PRAYERS & CHALLENGES

....

....

....

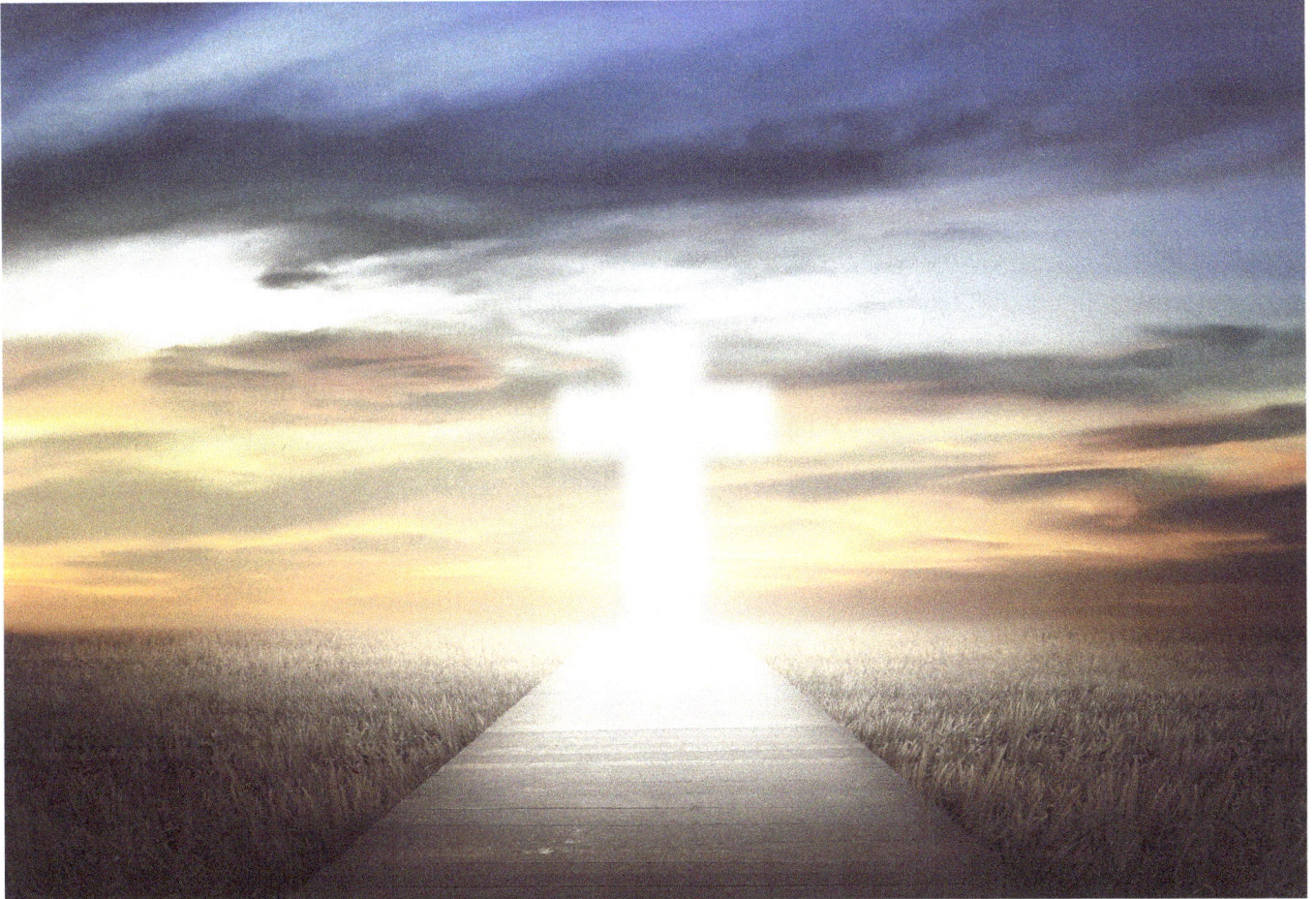

Intimacy with God

"Trust in the Lord with all thine heart; and lean not unto thine own understanding. In all thy ways acknowledge him, and he shall direct thy paths" (**Prov. 3:5, 6**).

Developing trust in God means learning to cling to Christ as your only hope of righteousness. God will work in your behalf when you do this. Picture yourself literally clinging to Christ in prayer. He is holding you up with His righteous right hand.

Have faith, but work; put your faith into action. This is the remedy for the habit you are trying to change. Bring all your life's habits into complete obedience to the laws of God and see Christ's righteousness complete the work in you. Christ meets you most of the way. He is only waiting for you to put forth your effort first in both asking and doing. He will give you the desire if you only ask.

DEVELOPING INTIMACY WITH GOD

THE CROSS—The cross was the ultimate act of love. The shadow of the cross is love. The love of God for you cannot be measured. In your affliction, Christ is working out your salvation. Be patient and pray for understanding. Bear your affliction cheerfully and if it is His will, He will soon lift the burden from you.

HIS RIGHTEOUSNESS—Many people are struggling to understand Christ's righteousness. Right now, I understand it to mean His righteous will, or His purity and goodness. We can do nothing about our filthy behavior, but He can take it and change it into His righteous behavior. We have no power on our own except to ask Him for help; then He does it for us and in us.

IT IS YOUR CHOICE—Everything that will happen to you in life is a result of your choices. The best way to choose is to ask Christ to help you. Always seek to find out what His way for you in each particular situation is, and follow it.

YOU CAN DO NOTHING ON YOU OWN— Stop the struggle. You cannot change yourself, but He can. Every morning, you can put on His robe of righteousness *with the hood*. It will cover you from your head to your feet. Acknowledge that you can do nothing, except through Christ who strengthens you (see Phil 4:13).

YOUR FAITH—According to Hebrews 11:1, "...Faith is the substance of things hoped for, the evidence of things not seen." Having faith in God is simply believing His promises for you and expecting them to come true.

Abiding faith puts aside personal feelings and selfish desires. If you abide in Christ, He will abide in you. Abiding is the act of walking humbly with the Lord and putting His promises into action on all occasions.

To abide in faith is to also believe that God will work out His own plans and purposes in your heart and life to purify your character. When you abide in faith, you rely and trust implicitly upon the faithfulness of God, and not on any earthly support.

PHYSICAL AWARENESS

My Current Health Assessment

1. Do you have a daily devotional time? Yes /No

2. If no, would you like to have one? Yes/No

3. Do you have difficulty in trusting the Lord with your problems? Yes/No/Sometimes

4. Do you suffer any remorse, guilt, worry, or fear? Yes/No

5. Do you believe that God has forgiven your sins? Yes/No

6. Do you struggle with knowing God's will for you? Yes/No

7. Do you have a spiritually strong immediate family? Yes/No

8. Do you have peace with God and people? Yes /No

9. Have you broken any vows or promises to God? Yes/No

10. If the Lord were to come today, from the life that you are currently living, would you be saved? *(please answer this question in your heart.)*

YOUR CHALLENGES ARE:

__to sit right up in bed when God calls to you in the morning.

__to immediately thank Him for another day.

__to take care of bathroom needs.

__to find a secret spot to pray and worship Him.

__to do a **SECOND MILE ACT** for someone:

__**to claim this promise:** *"Call unto me, and I will answer thee, and shew thee great and mighty things, which thou knowest not"* *(Jer. 33:3).*

RECIPE FOR THE DAY

20-MINUTE BISCUITS or BREAD

1 Tbsp. yeast

2 tsp. sugar/honey

½ cup warm water

¾ cup rolled oats

1 tsp salt

1 cup hot water

¼ cup oil

3 cups flour

PREHEAT oven to 375 degrees. Dissolve yeast in warm water and honey. Wait 5 minutes. At the same time, in another bowl, add oats, salt, and oil to the 1 cup of hot water, and let it sit for 5 minutes. Combine mixtures. Add enough flour to have a soft, but not sticky, dough. Let this sit for 10 minutes. Roll out dough and cut 1 inch thick. Place on baking sheet. Bake 15–20 minutes or until top is slightly brown. Enjoy!

MENTAL & MORAL AWARENESS

STEPS OF THE SANCTUARY PRAYER WALK

The story is told of a lady who was dying of cancer in the hospital and had only one month to live, so she asked God to reveal Himself to her in the best way before she died. He impressed her to study Him in the Sanctuary. She did, and ended up walking out of the hospital healed.

David says, "Thy way, O God, is in the sanctuary" (Ps. 77:13). Remember the three temples: the heavenly temple or sanctuary, the earthly temple (sanctuary) built by Moses, and the human temple (body).

LET US START WALKING

- ◆ **Open your hands upward** and in your mind; walk boldly to the throne of God to petition our heavenly Father for your needs and wants through the merits of Jesus Christ our Lord and Savior.

- ◆ In your mind, **enter into His Gates** with praise and thanksgiving *(Ps. 100:4 and Ps. 50:23)*.

- ◆ In the Old Testament, there was a gate to the sanctuary where they brought the lambs to be slain for their sins. Thankfully, we do not have to bring a lamb, because Jesus Christ the Lamb was slain for us from the foundation of the world *(Rev. 3:8)*.

WHAT DOES THE BIBLE SAY?

The Sanctuary

- • What happened on the Day of Atonement *(Lev. 16:33, 34)*?
- • What did the Old Testament sanctuary represent *(Heb. 9:9–12)*?
- • Who is our High Priest *(Heb. 8: 1–5)*?
- • How is sin to be removed from the heavenly sanctuary *(Heb. 9:23–25)*?

✓ *DAILY WELLNESS CHECK*

__Did I eat more fruits and vegetables today?

__Was I intimate with God today?

MY PRAYERS & CHALLENGES

....

....

....

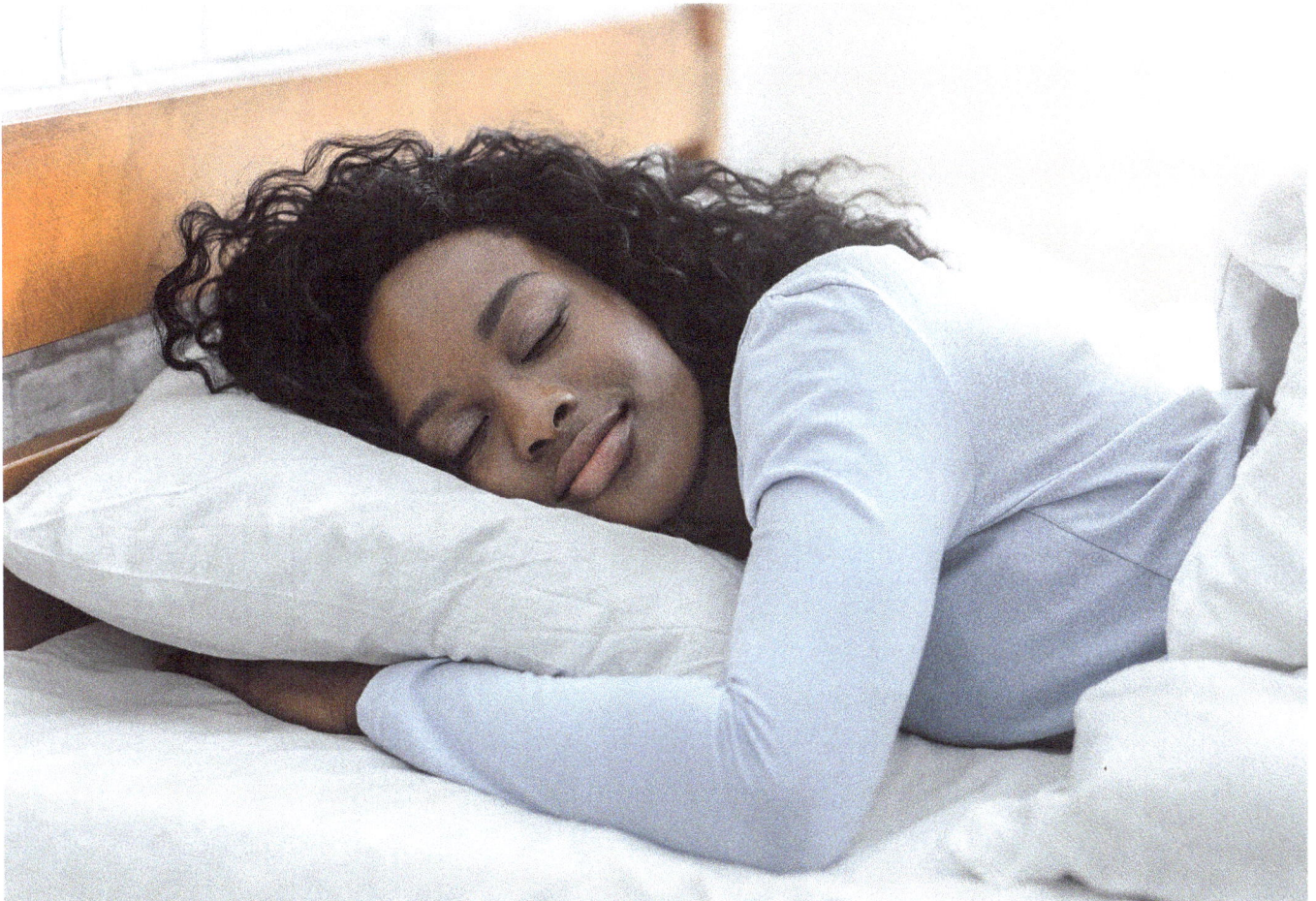

Sweet Sleep

"When thou liest down, thou shalt not be afraid: yea, thou shalt lie down, and thy sleep shall be sweet" (Prov. 3:24).

Scientists say that due to a lack of sleep, individuals are bad tempered and impatient on the road. They are constantly in a hurry and insensitive to others on the road; therefore, they develop "road rage" syndrome. There is also an increase of cranky employees, and more of them fall to sleep on the job. Due to a lack of sleep, mothers are going into depression more often.

"A factor that may play a part in road rage involves something that happens before we start our day—sleep. The National Sleep Foundation claims that a national epidemic of sleepiness can subject us to feelings of annoyance, resentment and anger. By getting more sleep at night, you can reduce your irritability and avoid some feelings associated with road rage" (Kruse 2018).

FACTS ABOUT REST

- Going to bed early can help control and maintain normal blood pressure.
- A lack of sleep contributes to obesity. This is due to an increase of stress and inflammation hormones.
- Staying awake late at night weakens the immune system.

PHYSICAL AWARENESS

My Current Health Assessment

1. What is your usual bedtime? _____
2. Do you wake up during the night? Yes/No/Sometimes
3. Do you snack before you go to bed? Yes/ No/Sometimes
4. Do you sleep with the lights on? Yes/No/Sometimes
5. Do you work the night or swing shift? Yes/No/Sometimes
6. Do you wake up early in the morning and find it difficult to get back to sleep? Yes/No/Sometimes
7. Do you take sleeping pills? Yes/No
8. Do you rest from labor at least one day per week? Yes/No

YOUR CHALLENGES ARE:

__to try and go to bed at the same time every night. The best time to fall asleep is between 9 and 10 pm.

__to keep the window slightly open.

__to do a **SECOND MILE ACT** for someone:

__**to claim this promise:** *"Come unto me…and I will give you rest"* (Matt. 11:28).

RECIPES FOR THE DAY

SPICY FRENCH FRIES

SCRUB potatoes and slice into ¼-inch thick pieces, like French fries. Place in a large sealable baggie and add a little oil, then salt, onion, garlic powder, paprika, and/or sweet basil.

SHAKE baggie for 30 seconds. Take potato slices out of baggie and then place on a cookie sheet sprinkled with oil. Bake for 40 minutes at 400 degrees. You can cover them to keep them moist while baking or uncover them for crispier fries.

SERVE with ketchup.

KETCHUP

1 can (8 oz.) tomato sauce

½ can (4 oz.) tomato paste

¼ cup honey or apple juice concentrate (or less)

¼ cup lemon juice

½ Tbsp. onion powder

½ tsp. paprika

½ tsp. sweet basil

¼ tsp. garlic powder

BLEND until smooth and refrigerate.

MENTAL & MORAL AWARENESS

STEPS OF THE SANCTUARY PRAYER WALK

◆ As you walk in your prayers to the throne of God, **approach the Altar of Burnt Offering.**

◆ Go to **His Altar of Burnt Offering** (Sacrifice) with repentance and confession of your sins. Plead for the blood of Christ to cover your sins (James 4:7–10 and Isa. 53).

◆ Let the Lord Jesus Christ put His priestly robe on you and then the censer of incense in your hands. Let Him draw you close to His side, holding your right hand with His right hand. It is a lover's embrace. Now pray. It is a wonderful scene to behold while on your knees. Picture yourself resting your head on His chest.

◆ **Remember to thank God that we do not have to sacrifice a lamb like in the Old Testament (Ex. 38:1–7). Jesus is the lamb.**

WHAT DOES THE BIBLE SAY?

Inspiration of the Bible

• What did Jesus say about Himself _(John 14:6)?_

• What is truth _(John 17:17)?_

• Where did the Bible come from _(2 Tim. 3:15, 16)?_

• What part did the Holy Spirit play _(2 Peter 1:21)?_

✓ _DAILY WELLNESS CHECK_

___Did I eat more fruits and vegetables today?_

___Was I intimate with God today?_

___Am I ready for bed on time today?_

MY PRAYERS & CHALLENGES

....

....

....

Day 4 Date _____

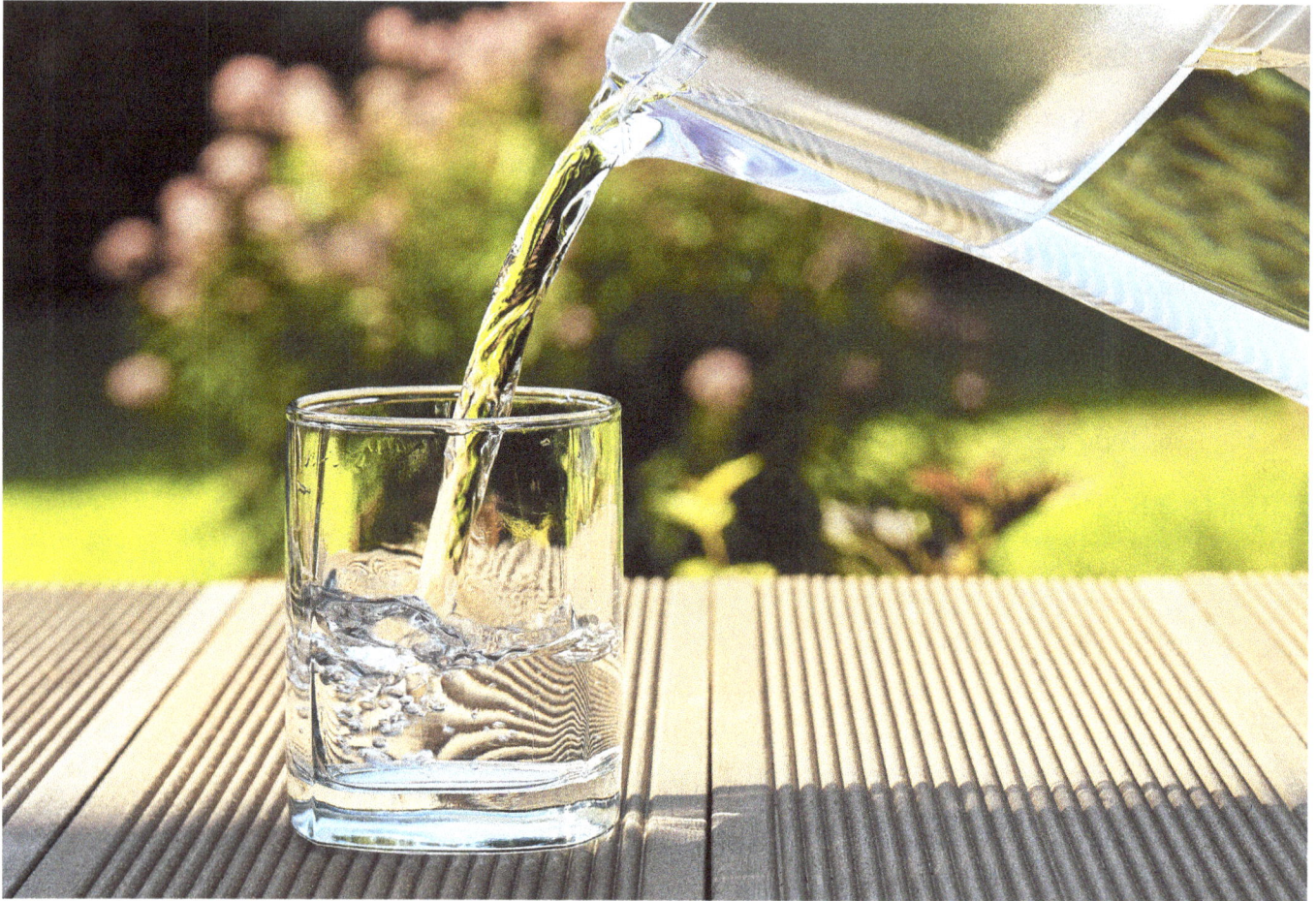

Soft Water

"And ye shall serve the Lord your God, and he shall bless thy bread, and thy water; and
I will take sickness away from the midst of thee" (Ex. 23:25).

Our bodies need water both on the inside and the outside. Water is by far the largest single component of the body, constituting 45–75% of total body mass, depending on age and gender (Tortora and Reynolds 2000, p. 957). Water has been used for the medical treatment of many diseases and is certainly used to prevent disease as well.

When water loss is greater than water gain, this results in dehydration. Some older people have constipation because they are not drinking enough water (Ferrell 2010, p. 490). It is vital that you increase the amount of water you drink! Kidney health is key to an adequate fluid level in the blood (p. 456). Hypertension (High Blood Pressure) is also affected by the amount of water consumed. Dr. Whitaker says, "Drink 15 glasses of water a day. Almost all the blood pressure medications mimic the effects of increased water intake. They usually do this by thinning the blood. Drink more water, and blood pressure will lower naturally" (p. 526).

FACTS ABOUT WATER

- Brain cells and kidneys are particularly sensitive to dehydration.

- The brain is between 70 and 85 percent water (Foster 1990, p. 84). Many people suffer headaches simply because they do not drink enough water, and they suffer from backache because the kidneys do not get enough water. It is said that drinking 1 glass of water every 10 minutes for 1 hour relieves most headaches (McNeilus 2010, p. 9).

- Water keeps the body temperature within a normal range.

- Our body cells' transportation of nutrients, elimination of waste, balance of chemicals in the body, production of digestive juices, and healthy action of the stomach and intestines, are all dependent upon water. "Dr. Hoffman says that if anything in the world can be called a Panacea, it is pure water. Water purifies the innumerable passages of the human body" (Paulien 1997, p. 98).

PHYSICAL AWARENESS

My Current Health Assessment

1. How many glasses of water do you drink per day? _____
2. What kind of water do you drink? _____
3. At what temperature do you drink your water? ___ Hot ___Cold ___Room temperature
4. Do you eat ice? Yes/No
5. How many glasses of juice do you drink per day? ____
6. How many cans/bottles of soda do you drink per day? ____
7. Circle the liquids you drink: tea, wine, alcohol, beer, soda, milk, vitamin water, ____
8. Do you drink with your meals? Yes/No
9. What color is your urine normally? ___clear ___slightly yellow ___yellow ___dark yellow

YOUR CHALLENGES ARE:

__to drink half your body weight in ounces of water (i.e., 160lbs/2=80. Drink 80 ounces of water each day).

__to drink water at room temperature.

__to give yourself a treat: **A SALT GLOW** (See the end of this chapter.)

__to do a **SECOND MILE ACT** for someone:

__**to claim this promise:** *"Beloved, if our heart condemn us not, then have we confidence toward God. And whatsoever we ask, we receive of him, because we keep his commandments, and do those things that are pleasing in his sight"* (1 John 3:21, 22).

RECIPES FOR THE DAY

BAKED OATMEAL

2 cups oats

¾ cups raisins

20 oz. unsweetened pineapple

1 tsp. salt

¼ cups coconut

¼ cups nuts

4–6 cups water

COMBINE all ingredients in given order. Bake for 1 hour at 350 degrees. Serves 6.

BAKED RICE

3 cups brown rice in a large, glass dish

7 cups water

½ to 1 Tbsp. onion power

½ tsp. thyme

Season with ocean salt to taste

COVER with aluminum foil and bake for 1 hour 20 minutes on 350 degrees. Turn stove off and let it stay in oven for another 10 minutes. You can store some in freezer bags for later meals.

MENTAL & MORAL AWARENESS

STEPS OF THE SANCTUARY PRAYER WALK

- ◆ **Walk to the His Laver of Washing.** Ask for cleansing (see Ps. 51). Ask the Father to cleanse you from old habits and attitudes (Ps. 51:7–12). Stay there until you have a sense of a newness and restoration.
- ◆ **In the Old Testament, the priest washes his feet and hands at the laver before they entered the Holy Place (Ex. 38:8).**

WHAT DOES THE BIBLE SAY?

Inspiration from the Bible

- Why was the Old Testament written *(Rom. 15:4)?*
- Did Jesus use the Old Testament to teach *(Luke 24:27)?*
- What can the words of Jesus do *(John 6:63)?*
- What will God's word do for your life *(Ps. 119:105)?*

✓ *DAILY WELLNESS CHECK*

__*Did I eat more fruits and vegetables today?*

__*Was I intimate with God today?*

__*Am I ready for bed on time today?*

__*Did I drink enough water today?*

MY PRAYERS & CHALLENGES

… …

… …

… …

HEALTHY TIDBITS:

The purposes and effects of **SALT GLOW** treatments are: to stimulate circulation, to increase nerve activity, to increase a sense of well-being and feelings of vitality, and to remove dead skin.

Salt Glow will benefit those with chronic indigestion, diabetes, sluggish circulation, weakened immune system that is prone to frequent colds, low blood pressure, and general weakness or low endurance.

If you are trying to stop smoking, it will make it easier to detox your body from the nicotine as you soak in a hot tub of water.

HOW TO DO A SALT GLOW: Place two cups of Epsom Salts in a bowl. Wet it slightly so it looks like snow. Do not let it dissolve. Then, stand in the shower and take some of the salts in your hand, and start rubbing your skin with strokes towards your heart. Some of the strokes should be in a circular motion. Rub the salts all over your body and even your face. Rinse off all the salts. You will feel like velvet because now you have washed off all the dead skin.

The salt glow is a stimulant type of special massage which can be used for a number of conditions. It is a very pleasant treatment if given properly; for epilepsy, general tonic, chronic illness of any kind, stimulant for muscles, nerves, or skin, cancer and other debilitation diseases (Thrash and Thrash, p. 74).

Typically, this method should not be used on the aged, or infants, or those with weak hearts or circulatory problems, because it so powerfully pumps the blood in and out of the body tissues. If there is any question, check first with your doctor.

A COLD SHOWER TREATMENT has a special tonic-like effect on the entire system. It stimulates the glandular system. It improves digestion and speeds up general metabolism. It will increase resistance to infections and colds if used regularly. It has a powerful influence on the central nervous system, on the brain, and on all the vital organs of the body. Scientists have discovered that water therapy can help the human body in a variety of ways (Ferrell and Cherne 2010, p. 216). It increases the blood count and has an electro-magnetic effect on the body, stimulating the flow of life energies and increasing the intake of oxygen to a remarkable degree.

Here is a tip on how to get well: When taking a hot bath or shower, you should finish with 20–60 seconds of cold water as a tonic and health boost. Another option is to alternate between very warm and very cold water, 3–7 times during one bath or shower. Do 1–3 minutes of warm water and 30–60 seconds of cold. Always finish with cold. Do this before bed at night so you can rest. You will be impressed with the results.

Friends suffering from Carpal Tunnel Syndrome, muscle pain, leg pain, swelling, and colds have told us that they had wonderful results by using these treatments.

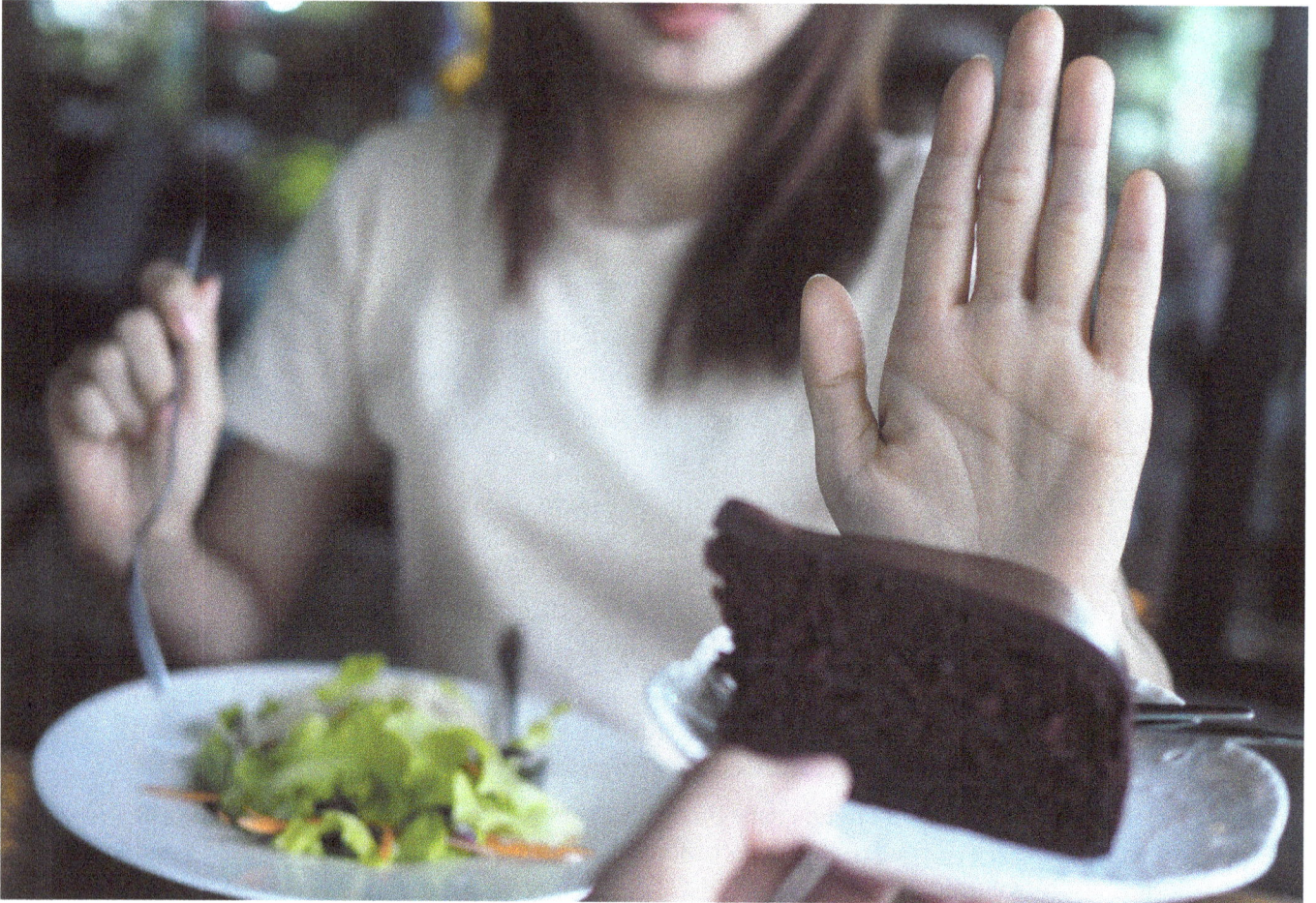

Temperance Always

"Whether therefore ye eat, or drink, or whatsoever ye do, do all to the glory of God" (1 Cor. 10:31).

Life seems to be a balancing act, so many do's and don'ts. A good rule to live by is to completely avoid those things that are harmful, and always be temperate (balanced) with the things that are good.

FACTS ON TEMPERANCE

- Perfect health is connected to perfect circulation, and this cannot be done without good blood (Ferrell and Cherne, p. 74).

- To achieve maximum health, we should eat properly and eliminate all alcoholic beverages, coffee, tobacco, and other damaging drugs.

- Avoid overworking the digestive system by not eating foods that are too hot or too cold. The stomach has to work hard to bring food to a proper temperature for digestion.

- Controlling the appetite will give moral and physical victory over many vices. Cutting back on meat-eating, tea, coffee, and cola drinking will clear up a multitude of problems and avoid even more. Peptic ulcers and osteoporosis will be avoided or eliminated. Diseases of the breast, the prostate, the ovary and the bladder are also diminished.

- Most cancers start in the stomach and go throughout the blood stream; this can be greatly avoided if meat eating is eliminated or reduced. Nervousness, anxiety, tremors, dizziness, sleep and memory disturbances, headaches, and depression will be alleviated if these items are absent from the lifestyle.

- To help remove these problems, drink your required amount of water each day. Bathe several times a day to remove body waste from the skin. Exercise out in the fresh air and sunshine. Practice deep breathing and proper posture. Eat a simple, healthful diet consisting of fruits, vegetables, whole grains, nuts, and seeds. Abstain from all beverages containing alcohol or caffeine.

PHYSICAL AWARENESS

My Current Health Assessment

1. What is your current occupation? _____

2. Do you smoke/use tobacco products in any form (i.e. chewing tobacco)? Yes/No

3. Did you use tobacco in the past? Yes/No. If so, how much and for how long? _____

4. Do you use alcohol in any form? Yes/No. If so, how much and for how long? _____

5. Do you ingest caffeine in any form? Yes/ No. Circle: coffee, teas, colas, energy drinks, other_____

6. Do you overeat? Yes/No/Sometimes

7. Do you finish your meal in under twenty minutes? Yes/No/Sometimes

8. Do you snack between meals? Yes/No/Sometimes

9. Do you eat sugary foods? Yes/No/Sometimes

10. Circle your leisure activities (watching TV, reading, sports, dancing, board games other_____)

11. How much time do you spend a day doing leisure activities? _____

12. Do you overwork? Yes/No/Sometimes

13. Please list any addictions _____

14. Have you been involved with substance abuse? Yes/No. List: _____

15. Do you read (circle) novels, science fiction, pornography, fashion, magazines?

16. How much time do you spend a day on the computer with games, business, etc.?_____

YOUR CHALLENGES ARE:

__to stay away from things that are bad.

__to be moderate with the good things you eat, drink, and do.

__to do a **SECOND MILE ACT** for someone:

__**to claim this promise:** *"Fear thou not; for I am with thee: be not dismayed; for I am thy God: I will strengthen thee; yea, I will help thee; yea, I will uphold thee with the right hand of my righteousness" (Isa. 41:10).*

RECIPE FOR THE DAY

MUSTARD

¾ cup lemon juice

¼ cup flour

½ tsp. onion powder

1½ tsp. garlic powder

1½ tsp. turmeric

½ tsp. salt

2 Tbsp. water

⅓ cup oil

BLEND all ingredients except the oil. Cook in a small pot on medium heat until it thickens. Cool and return to blender, then add oil in a thin stream while blending.

MENTAL & MORAL AWARENESS

STEPS OF THE SANCTUARY PRAYER WALK

◆ After being washed ask Christ to clothe you with **His robe of righteousness.** Have faith that His righteous will can do all things in you through His strength (Phil. 4:13).

◆ **While in prayer, contemplate how true the Word of God (His promises) has proven itself to you. As you put on the breast plate of righteousness, think of the good things that you know need to be done. Then think of sharing the gospel with someone today, if not by word, then just by a peaceful smile. The helmet of salvation should make you think about Yeshua's sacrifice to save you. And finally, the Sword of the Spirit, the Word of God, comforts, protects, and defends you (Eph. 6:13–18).**

WHAT DOES THE BIBLE SAY?

Second Coming

- What promise did Jesus give *(John 14:1–3)*?
- How will Christ come *(Acts 1:9–11)*?
- Who will see Him come *(Rev. 1:7)*?
- Is Jesus a real person *(Luke 24:36–43, 50)*?

✓ *DAILY WELLNESS CHECK*

__*Did I eat more fruits and vegetables today?*

__*Was I intimate with God today?*

__*Am I ready for bed on time today?*

__*Did I drink enough water today?*

__*Did I overdo anything today?*

MY PRAYERS & CHALLENGES

… …

… …

… …

HEALTHY TIDBITS

Top 10 Food Additives to Avoid, by Dr. Mercola (2010):

Food additives have been used to enhance the appearance and flavor of food and prolong shelf life. They help ease processing packaging and storage and give it long shelf life. These additives make the food artificial, which has serious consequences to your health.

ARTIFICIAL SWEETENERS: like **Aspartame (also known as** NutraSweet® or Equal®), is known to erode intelligence and affect short-term memory.

HIGH FRUCTOSE CORN SYRUP: is the number one source of calories in America, and keeps you from knowing when to stop eating.

MONOSODIUM GLUTAMATE (MSG): keeps you from feeling satisfied, so you overeat.

TRANS FAT: is used to deep fry foods, causing cholesterol, which can lead to heart attacks and strokes.

COMMON FOOD DYES: are found in sodas, fruit juices, and salad dressings; can cause behavior issues and low IQs.

Blue #1 and Blue #2: is found in cereal and sports drinks.

Red dye #3 (Red #40, a more current dye)**:** is found in ice cream, candy, cherry pie.

Yellow #6 and yellow Tartrazine: is found in American cheese, candy, carbonated beverages.

SODIUM SULFITE: negatively affects airways and is found in wine and dried fruit.

SODIUM NITRATE/SODIUM NITRITE: can be found in cured meats, like hot dogs, and negatively affects the blood.

BHA and BHT: Affects brain and is found in chips.

SULFUR DIOXIDE: destroys vitamins B and E. This is found in beer, potato chips, soft drinks, and juices.

POTASSIUM BROMATE: is found in bread and can cause cancer in animals.

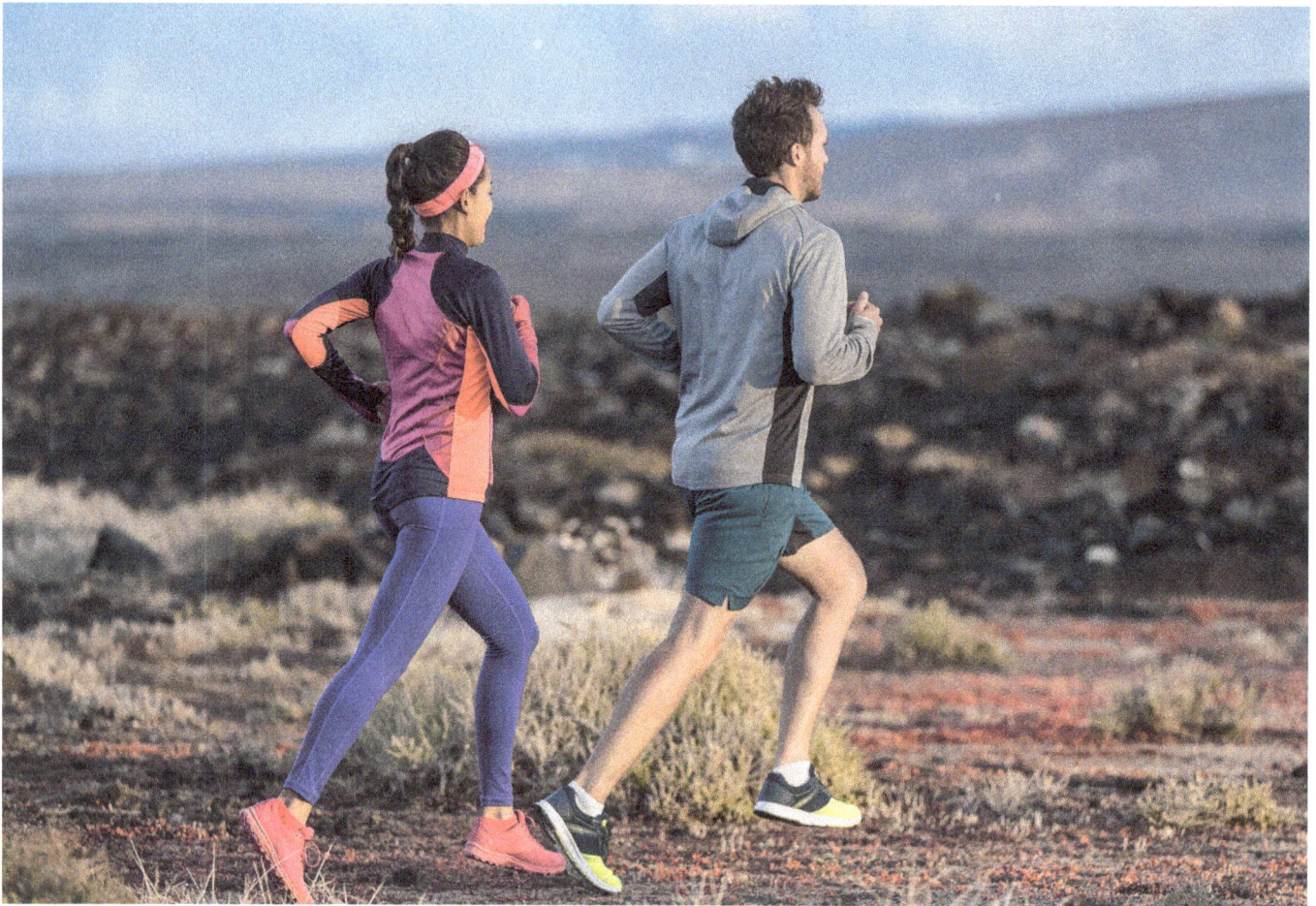

Exercise Daily

"There is nothing better for a man, than that he should eat and drink, and that he should make his soul enjoy good in his labour. This also I saw, that it was from the hand of God" (Eccles. 2:24).

"If you exercise every day and get your heart rate up just a few times a week, giving it a bit extra when you run, bike or swim, your body will get healthier than if you change your diet in the hope that you'll lose weight" (Hoffman 2012).

Others say, "The benefits of good nutrition are the same as exercise, making the two together a powerful recipe for good health" (Kueppers 2015)!

Remember what God had Adam and Eve do while in the garden, and continue doing when they were out of the garden? Their work was to train the vines, and after sin, to till the earth. Movement of the body and its organs gives strength and vigor, while inactivity leads to decay and death.

FACTS ABOUT EXERCISE

- Exercise is one of the most frequently prescribed therapies for both health and the healing of disease (Vina 2012).
- Perfect health depends on perfect circulation. Good circulation depends a large degree upon the muscle tone of the body.
- Walking and gardening are the best exercises.
- Exercising for thirty minutes per day, and at least three to four times per week, maintains perfect health.
- Walking sixty minutes every day aids in recovering from disease, to perfect health.

PHYSICAL AWARENESS

My Current Health Assessment

1. How many times a week do you exercise? _____

2. How many minutes per day do you exercise? _____

3. How would you rate your exercise?

_____Mild _____Moderate _____Vigorous

4. How do you feel after you exercise? _____

5. Are you in any pain during exercise? Yes/ No

YOUR CHALLENGES ARE:

__to walk for at least 10–20 minutes after breakfast or lunch, or even before bedtime.

__to try and get an hour of exercise of any kind daily, especially if you have a health issue.

__to do a **SECOND MILE ACT** for someone:

__**to claim this promise:** *"…Thine health shall spring forth speedily"* (Isa. 58:8).

RECIPE FOR THE DAY

OATMEAL SAUSAGE PATTIES

2 cups water

1 cup chopped onion

1 Tbsp. salt OR 3 Tbsp. soy sauce

2 tsp. maple syrup or honey

2 tsp. onion powder

½ tsp. garlic powder

1 tsp. Italian seasoning

1 tsp. sage/thyme or both

1 tsp. parsley flakes

1 cup pecan or walnut meal

2 cups quick oatmeal

BOIL all except nut meal and oatmeal. While boiling, add quick oats and nut meal. Turn off stove and stir to thicken. Cool, and then FORM into patties, and bake at 350 degrees on pre-oiled cookie sheet for 15–20 minutes. Flip over and bake for another 10 minutes. ENJOY!!!

MENTAL & MORAL AWARENESS

STEPS OF THE SANCTUARY PRAYER WALK

◆ **It is good to also ask the Lord to guard the avenues to your soul at this time. Your ears, eyes, nose, taste, and touch.**

◆ **Philippians 4:4–7 says, "Rejoice in the Lord always: and again I say, Rejoice. Let your moderation be known unto all men. The Lord is at hand. Be careful for nothing; but in every thing by prayer and supplication with thanksgiving let your request be made known unto God. And the peace of God, which passeth all understanding, shall keep your hearts and minds through Christ Jesus."**

◆ **Philippians 4:8 is wonderful to repeat in the prayer. "Whatsoever things are true, whatsoever things are honest, whatsoever things are just , whatsoever things are pure, whatever things are lovely, whatsoever things are of good report; if there be any virtue, and if there be any praise, think on these things."**

WHAT DOES THE BIBLE SAY?

Second Coming

- Why will Christ come *(Matt. 24:30, 31)*?
- What reward will Christ give *(Rev. 22:12)*?
- When will Christ come *(Matt. 24:36)*?
- What happens to those who are unprepared *(Rev. 6:14–17)*?
- What should we do now *(Matt. 24:37–44)*?

✓ *DAILY WELLNESS CHECK*

__*Did I eat more fruits and vegetables today?*

__*Was I intimate with God today?*

__*Am I ready for bed on time today?*

__*Did I drink enough water today?*

__*Did I overdo anything today?*

__*Did I exercise today?*

MY PRAYERS & CHALLENGES

....

....

....

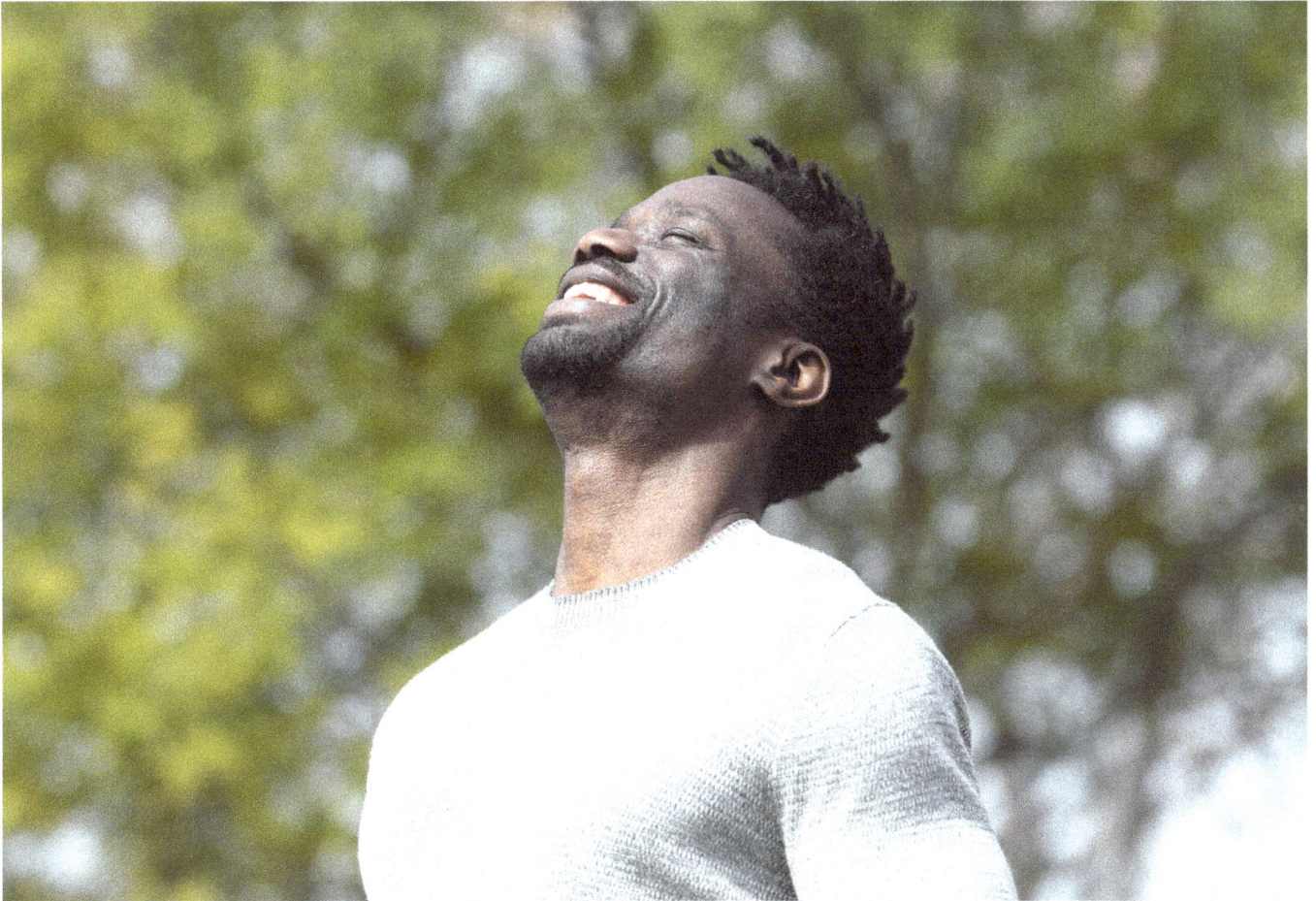

Pure, Fresh Air

"And the Lord God formed man of the dust of the ground, and breathed into his nostrils the breath of life; and man became a living soul" (Gen. 2:7).

The first thing we do when we move into a new or old house is to open the windows to let the fresh air in. The first thing we do when we enter this world is to gasp for air.

FACTS ABOUT PURE, FRESH AIR

- All nature depends on air.

- Air is the most vital element for man and animals. One may live for a week without food, or three days without water, but deprived of air, he will perish within minutes.

- The human body must have oxygen; each of its 100 trillion cells must receive steady, fresh supplies to survive.

- Every day you take more than 17,000 breaths to keep your body fueled.
- The heart sends blood to the lungs, where it drops off carbon dioxide for elimination and picks up fresh oxygen for delivery to every cell in the body.

PHYSICAL AWARENESS

My Current Health Assessment

1. Where do you live? City/Suburbs/Country

2. Do you sleep with your windows open? Yes/No

3. Do you open your windows and doors daily to air out the home? Yes/No

4. Do you live or work in a smoky place? Yes/No

5. Do you have live plants in your home? Yes/No

YOUR CHALLENGES ARE:

__to do deep breathing exercises every day.

__to keep the bedroom windows open at night.

__to air out the house for 10–20 minutes in the morning.

__to do a **SECOND MILE ACT** for someone:

__**to claim this promise:** *"...by whose stripes ye were healed"* (1 Peter 2:24).

RECIPE FOR THE DAY

SCRAMBLED TOFU or 'EGGS'

1 pack tofu

½ cup chopped onion

½ cup chopped sweet pepper

1 tsp. garlic powder

1 tsp. salt

1 tsp. turmeric

1 tsp. sweet basil

1 tsp. paprika

¼ cup yellow yeast flakes

SAUTE onions and peppers in a little oil or water. Crush tofu separately, and then add it, and other ingredients, to the sautéed onions. Stir, cover, and cook on low to medium heat until hot, and look yellow like eggs. ENJOY!

MENTAL & MORAL AWARENESS

STEPS OF THE SANCTUARY PRAYER WALK

- ◆ Go to **His lampstand of the Holy Spirit** and ask for your daily baptism with **His Holy Spirit.** Ask for His Spirit of wisdom, understanding, knowledge, discernment, counsel, fear of God, and power (Isa. 11:2–4).
- ◆ Ask Him to give you His faith, virtue, knowledge, temperance, patience, godliness, brotherly kindness, and love (2 Peter 1:4–11).

◆ **Ask for His love that is found in 1 Corinthians 13:4–8. (Read and memorize it.)**

◆ **Ask for and claim His fruit of the Spirit (Gal. 5:23, 24). Make this part of your prayer.**

WHAT DOES THE BIBLE SAY?

Signs of the Times

- What question did His disciples ask Jesus *(Matt. 24:1–3)?*
- What sign did Jesus give first *(Matt. 24:6)?*
- Name 3 other signs in verse 7 *(Matt. 24:7).*
- What condition will people be in the last days *(2 Tim. 3:1–5)?*
- How will Satan deceive many *(1 Tim. 4:1, 2)?*

✓ *DAILY WELLNESS CHECK*

__*Did I eat more fruits and vegetables today?*

__*Was I intimate with God today?*

__*Am I ready for bed on time today?*

__*Did I drink enough water today?*

__*Did I overdo anything today?*

__*Did I exercise today?*

__*Am I taking deep breaths today?*

MY PRAYERS & CHALLENGES

………

………

………

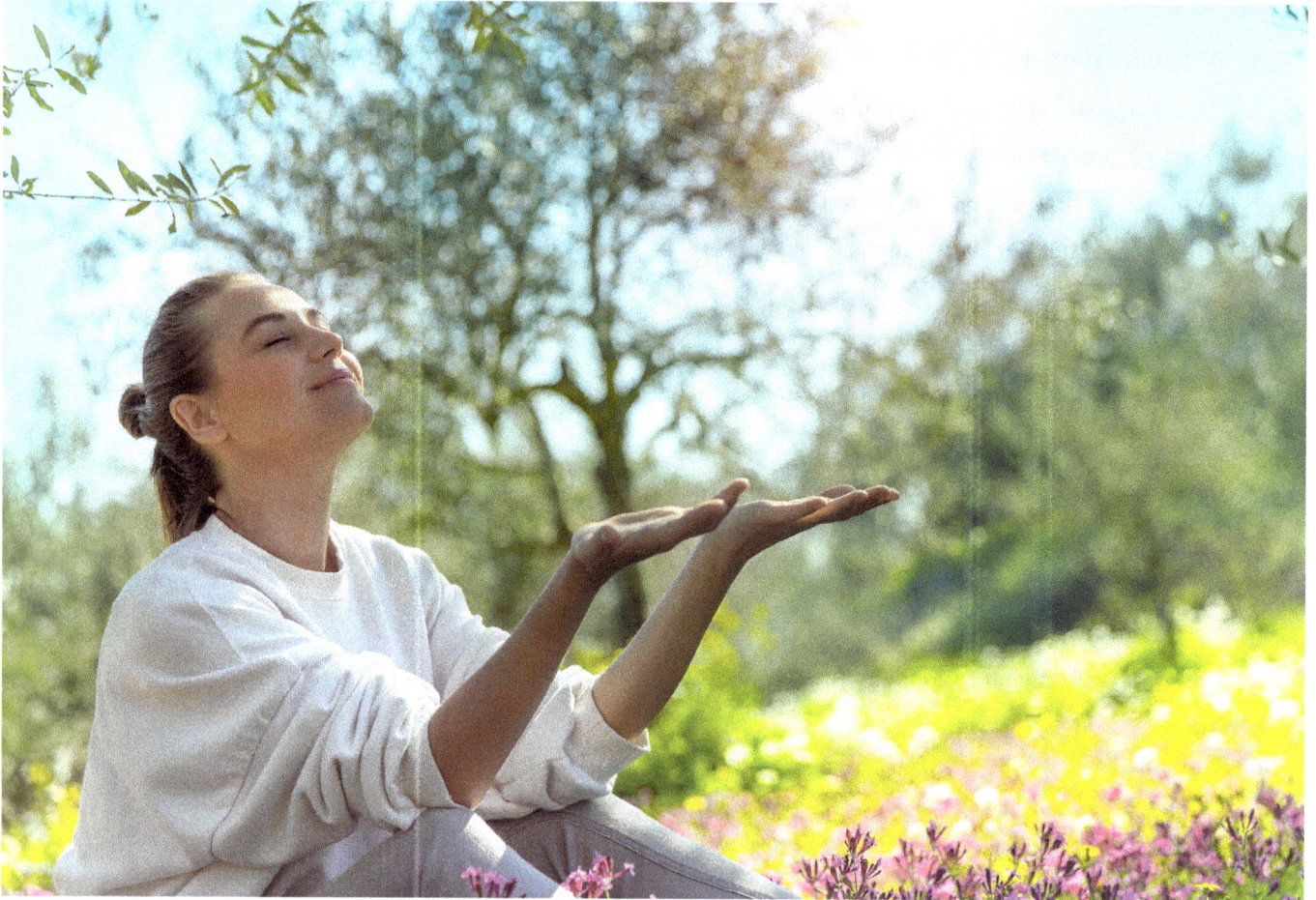

Sunlight

"Truly the light is sweet, and a pleasant thing it is for the eyes to behold the sun" (Eccles. 11:7).

Sunshine is sometimes thought to be bad, but it is very essential for better health. Sunshine converts the cholesterol under your skin into vitamin D. This vitamin D then goes to the bones and releases your calcium, which then takes all your vitamins into the body for optimum health.

FACTS ABOUT SUNLIGHT: How much is enough?

- Start with 10–15 minutes exposure to the face and hands daily, then gradually increase it to 30–45 minutes daily. The body will store the vitamin D for over a week.

- Darker skinned individuals need at least 30 minutes a day, and lighter skinned individuals need at least 15 minutes.

- The best times to avoid excessive sun exposure are before 10 a.m. and after 4 p.m. ("Sun Safety" 2012).
- When outdoors, wear protective clothing and a wide brimmed hat. Light cotton cloth allows the skin to absorb some of the sun's rays.

PHYSICAL AWARENESS

My Current Health Assessment

1. How many hours of sun do you get per day? _____
2. Do you frequently wear short sleeves in the sun? Yes/No
3. Do you use sun block? Yes/No/Sometimes
4. Do you have any abnormal sensitivity to the sun naturally, or due to any medications? Yes/No
5. Do you take vitamin D supplements? Yes/No

YOUR CHALLENGES ARE:

__to be in sun before 10 a.m. and after 4 p.m.

__to wear protective clothing and a wide brimmed hat when outdoors.

__to wear light cotton clothing outdoors because they allow the skin to absorb some of the sun's rays.

__to do a **SECOND MILE ACT** for someone:

__**to claim this promise:** *"…I have seen his ways, and will heal him: I will lead him also, and restore comforts unto him and to his mourners. I create the fruit of the lips; peace, peace to him that is a far off, and to him that is near, saith the Lord; I will heal him"* (Isa. 57:18, 19).

RECIPE FOR THE DAY

SHEILA'S SPECIAL GRANOLA

3 cups quick oats

1 cup oil

6 cup rolled oats

½ cup water

1 ½ cups unsweetened coconut

1 cup fruit juice

1 cup sunflower seeds

¼ cup honey or molasses

½ cup flax seeds

1 tsp. salt

1 cup coarsely chopped walnuts

1 Tbsp. vanilla

MIX dry ingredients in a large bowl. Then, add the liquid ingredients and mix well (using hands). Place in pans. Bake at 250 degrees for 1–2 hours, stirring after 30 minutes. Or, bake at 150–200 degrees overnight if desired (approx. 6–8 hours). Add dry fruit like raisins and pineapple after cooling, but before storing

MENTAL & MORAL AWARENESS

STEPS OF THE SANCTUARY PRAYER WALK

◆ The **Lampstand** represents the **Holy Spirit.** In the Old Testament (Ex. 37:17–24), this lampstand was made of solid gold and was always lit. This represents the consistent presence of the Holy Spirit in our lives.

◆ It is the presence of the Holy Spirit that is in our lives as the representative of Jesus Christ here on earth.

◆ **He is our comforter and the Spirt of Truth (John 14:16, 17, 26).**

WHAT DOES THE BIBLE SAY?

Signs of the Times

• What did Daniel predict about the end of time *(Dan. 12:4)?*

• Will everybody believe these signs *(2 Peter 3:3–5)?*

• What work remains to be done *(Matt. 24:14)?*

• What should be our attitude to all these things *(Luke 21:25–28)?*

✓ *DAILY WELLNESS CHECK*

__*Did I eat more fruits and vegetables today?*

__*Was I intimate with God today?*

__*Am I ready for bed on time today?*

__*Did I drink enough was today?*

__*Did I overdo anything today?*

__*Did I exercise today?*

__*Am I taking deep breaths today?*

__*Did I get enough sunshine today?*

MY PRAYERS & CHALLENGES

....

....

....

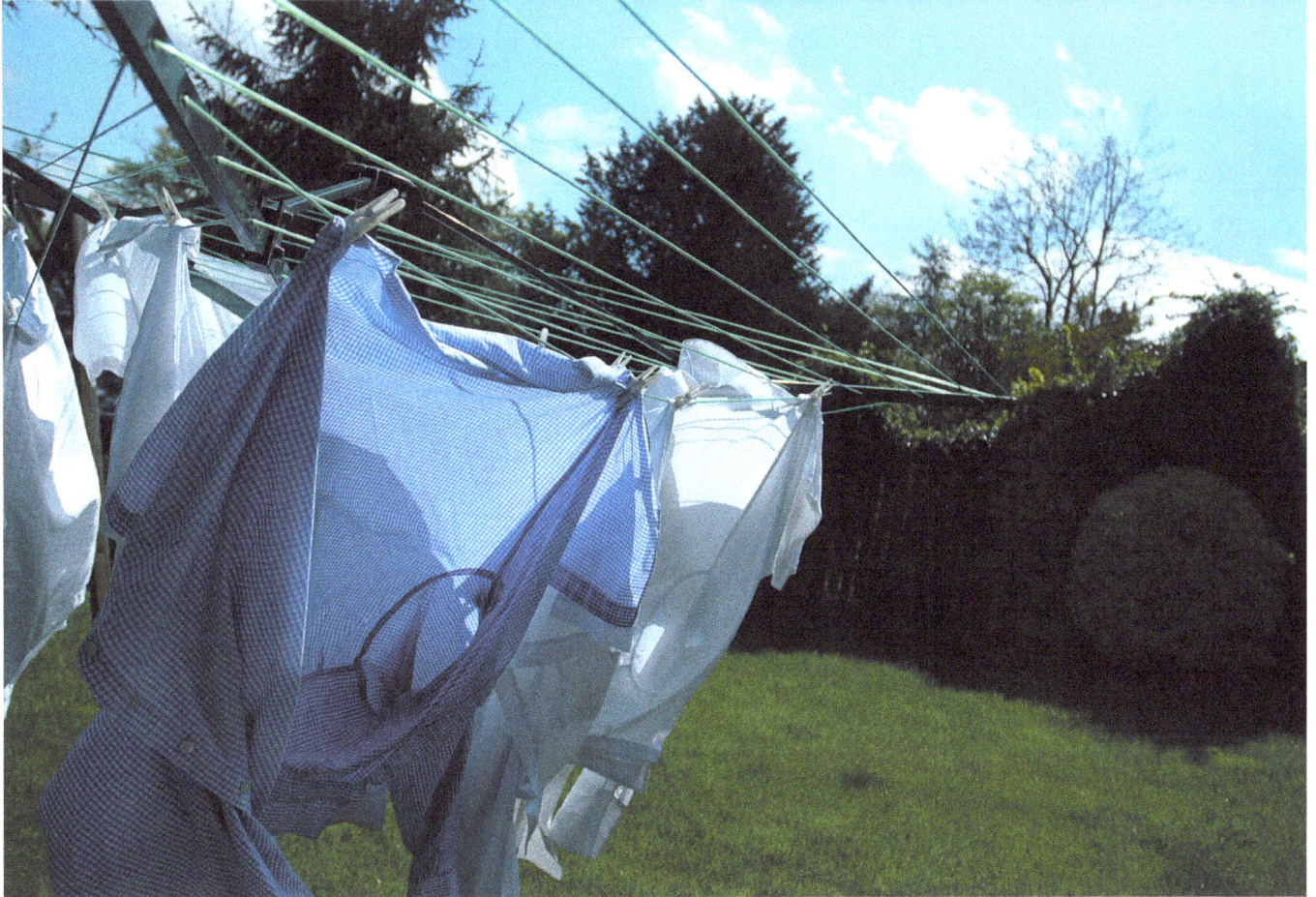

Wearing Clothes to Promote Health

"…that women adorn themselves in modest apparel, with shamefacedness and sobriety; not with broided hair, or gold, or pears, or costly array; But (which becometh women professing godliness) with good works" (1 Tim. 2:9, 10).

FACTS ABOUT WEARING HEALTHY CLOTHES

- It is best to wear clothing made out of natural fibers like cotton, wool, linen, and silk because they are more breathable, meaning they allow the air to circulate better on your skin.

- Dress and self-esteem are also intimately related. A person with high self-esteem is less likely to cheat on examinations. Stability and character are judged by dress, even your own self-judgment.

- Choose light colors, which reflect the heat and thus keep the body cool.

- Improper clothing causes both mental and physical disability.

PHYSICAL AWARENESS

My Current Health Assessment

1. Would you say that your dress is healthful and modest? Yes/No

2. Do you wear clothes (bra) too tight? Yes/No

3. Do you remember feeling cold when your arms and legs were exposed recently? Yes/No

YOUR CHALLENGES ARE:

__to look in your closet to see if you have cotton and linen clothes. They breathe better.

__to wear clothes with sleeves to the elbow or wrist.

__to wear clothes that are not tight fitting, so you can breathe better.

__to do a **SECOND MILE ACT** for someone:

__**to claim this promise:** *"...He shall teach you all things, and bring all things to your remembrance"* (John 14:26).

RECIPES FOR THE DAY

RAW VEGETABLE SOUP

BLEND until smooth and add 1–2 cups of hot boiled potato, including its water, with a variety of fresh vegetables. Add spices and salt to taste.

LENTIL, YELLOW or GREEN SPLIT PEA SOUP

BOIL beans for 20 minutes. Change water and boil for 1 hour with a medium chopped onion, add other ingredients like potatoes, carrots, spices, etc., for another hour or until done.

MENTAL & MORAL AWARENESS

STEPS OF THE SANCTUARY PRAYER WALK

◆ Now we will go to the **table of shewbread** or **the table of His presence.** The two stacks of bread represent Christ and His Father, and the Word of God.

◆ In our worship, we need to read the word of God, or eat of His flesh (see John 6:26–58). Partake of the body of Christ through the Word. Meditate on the words He gives you each morning from the Bible. They will become part of your plans for the day.

◆ **The table of shewbread stood on the north. With its ornamental crown, it was overlaid with pure gold. Each Sabbath, the priest arranged twelve cakes, sprinkled with frankincense, into two piles (Ex. 37:10–16).**

WHAT DOES THE BIBLE SAY?

Heaven

• Where did Jesus go after leaving *(John 14:1–3)*?

• What promise was made to the sheep *(Matt. 25:34)*?

• What did Abraham look for *(Heb. 11:10)*?

• Describe the Holy City *(Rev. 21:10–19)*.

• What will life be like in Heaven *(Isa. 33:24)*?

✓ *DAILY WELLNESS CHECK*

__Did I eat more fruits and vegetables today?

__Was I intimate with God today?

__Am I ready for bed on time today?

__Did I drink enough today?

__Did I overdo anything today?

__Did I exercise today?

__Am I taking deep breaths today?

__Did I get enough sunshine today?

__Did I dress appropriately today?

MY PRAYERS & CHALLENGES

....

....

....

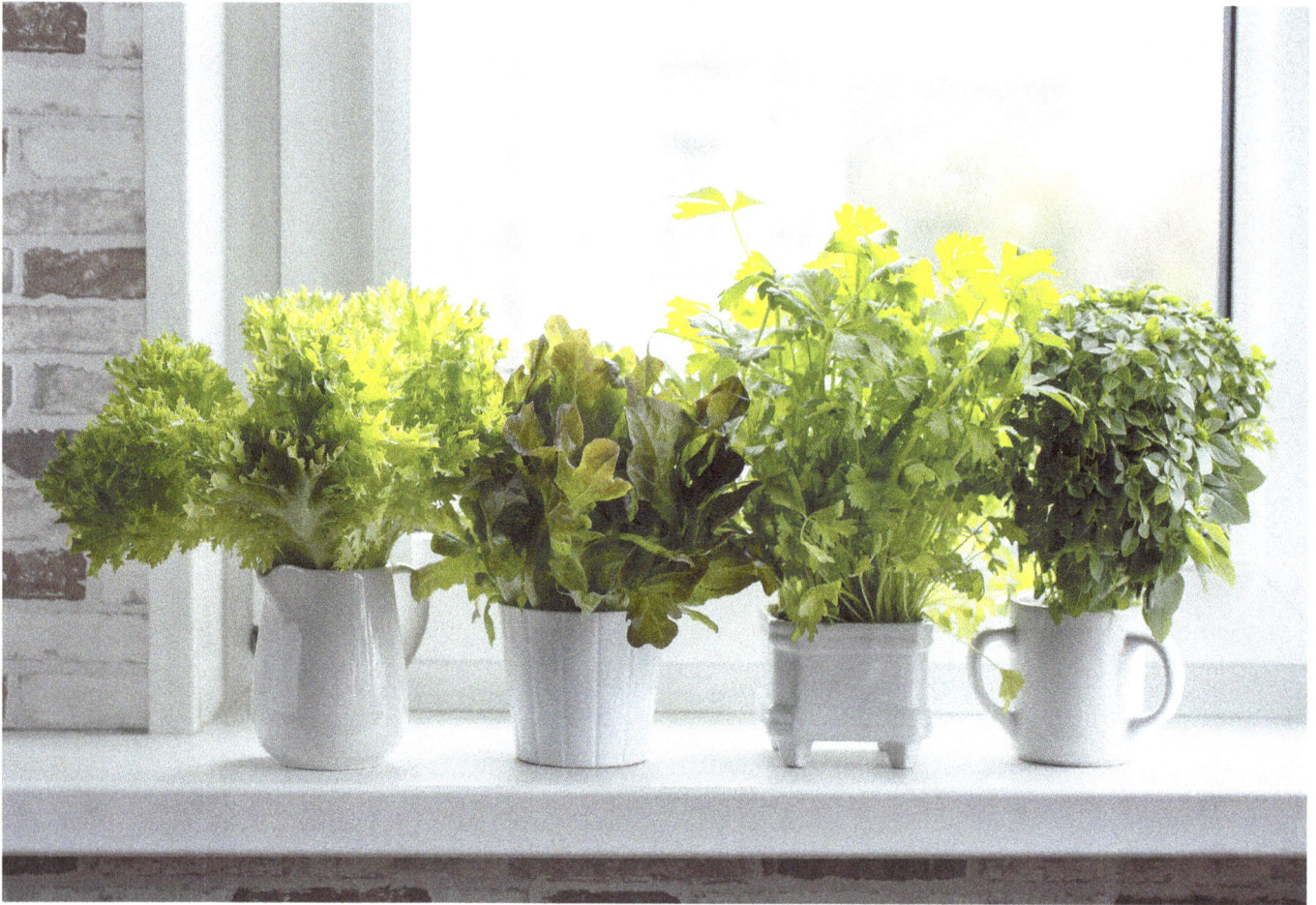

Physical Awareness

THE COLON CONNECTION

The colon is looked upon as the main source of human misery and suffering—mentally, physically and morally. "The warning 'Death begins in the colon,' has been ascribed to Dr. Bernard Jensen, D.C. who, in some circles, is referred to as the "Father of Colonics" (Lucas 2014). "Accumulating evidence suggests that gut bacteria play critical roles in maintaining human health in many aspects. Gut microbiota dysbiosis (parasites living in gut) may lead to a number of diseases, including gastrointestinal disorders, obesity, cardiovascular diseases, allergy and central nervous system-related diseases" (Wang 2018).

The colon is a sewage system, but by neglect and abuse it becomes a cesspool. When it is clean and normal then we are well and happy. Let it stagnate (become constipated) and it will diffuse the poisons into the blood, poisoning the brain and nervous system so that we become mentally depressed and irritable. It will poison the heart so that we are weak and listless. It will poison the lungs so that the breath is foul. It will poison the digestive organs so that we are distressed and bloated. It will poison the blood so that the skin is sallow and unhealthy.

In other words, every organ of the body becomes poisoned, and we age prematurely. We will look and feel old. Our joints become stiff and painful. Our eyes become dull and our sluggish brain overtakes us, and the pleasure of living is gone. What an awful experience, but there is hope: **Find what food causes you to go to the bathroom easily and eat it periodically.**

YOUR CHALLENGES ARE:

__to soak 4–6 prunes in natural salt water and lemon juice overnight, then eat them the next day.

__to eat more fiber fruit daily.

__to drink your proper amount of water daily.

__to exercise daily, even if you just march in place for 4 to 7 times, 7 minutes each time.

__to sit on the toilet within 5–10 minutes after you eat your meals.

__to do a **SECOND MILE ACT** for someone:

__**to claim this promise:** *"And take heed to yourselves, lest at any time your hearts be overcharged with surfeiting (overeating), and drunkenness (alcoholism), and cares of this life…"* (Luke 21:34).

HERBS and HOW TO USE THEM IN COOKING

ANISE—Cinnamon substitute, cookies, cakes, applesauce, rye bread

BASIL—Tomatoes, tomato sauce, corn chowder, squash, stew, scrambled tofu

BAY LEAVES—Tomatoes, soups, beans, stews

CARAWAY SEED—Breads, pumpernickel, cookies, cabbage salad, beets, rye

CARDAMON—Whole for pickling, Ground for bun breads, pastry, coffee cakes

CELERY SEED—Salads, salad dressings; Ground for tomato juice and flakes for soups, stews, and stuffing

CHIVES—All salads, scalloped (Hurd, Frank and Hurd, Rosalie. "A Good Cook…TEN TALENTS" 1968, pp. 164-166)

MENTAL & MORAL AWARENESS

STEPS OF THE SANCTUARY PRAYER WALK

◆ The next step is the **Altar of Intersession.** Here is where you pray for others. We become intercessors. This is a very important step, because we need to do what our Savior is constantly doing now, which is interceding for us as our High Priest (Heb. 7:25; 8:1, 2.)

YOUR PRAYER FOR THE SICK

Pray this while you are in the presence of the sick:

Lord, You know every secret of the soul.

You are acquainted with _____ (name).

If therefore, it is for Your glory and good for this affliction to pass, we ask, in the name of Jesus, that _____ (name) be restored to health.

If it is not Your will, we ask that Your grace may comfort, and Your presence sustain them in their sufferings.

May the God of peace sanctify you wholly; I pray to God for your whole Spirit and soul and body be preserved, blameless to the coming of our Lord Jesus Christ.

In the name of Yeshua, who is also called Jesus, Amen.

WHAT DOES THE BIBLE SAY?

Heaven

- Why will Heaven be such a happy place *(Rev. 21:4)*.

- Will we worship in Heaven *(Isa. 66:21, 23)?*

- Who will be in Heaven *(Matt. 24:31)?*

- Will we know our loved ones there *(1 Cor. 13:12)?*

- What must we do to make sure of a place in Heaven *(Rev. 22:14)?*

✓ *DAILY WELLNESS CHECK*

__Did I eat more fruits and vegetables today?

__Was I intimate with God today?

__Am I ready for bed on time today?

__Did I drink enough water today?

__Did I overdo anything today?

__Did I exercise today?

__Am I taking deep breaths today?

__Did I get enough sunshine today?

__Did I dress appropriately today?

MY PRAYERS & CHALLENGES

....

....

....

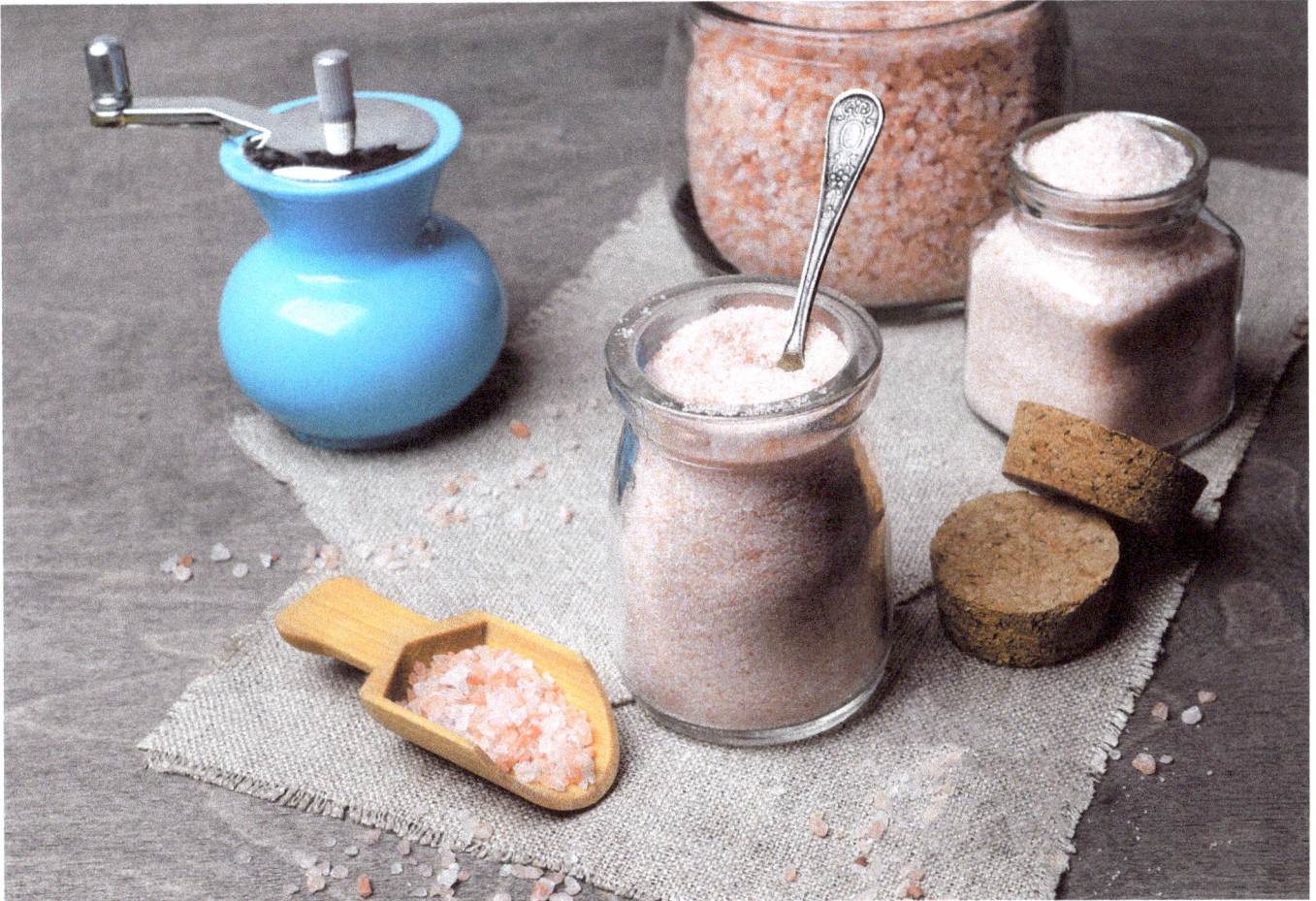

Physical Awareness

MORE ABOUT HEALTHY FOODS

Eat a variety of fruits, grains, vegetables, legumes (beans), seeds, and nuts prepared in a simple tasty way. Eating a varied selection of natural plant foods will furnish all the nutrients the body requires. For maximum health and energy, the body needs a low fat, moderate protein, high carbohydrate diet with sufficient micronutrients and fiber.

GOD'S FOODS RESTORE

THE BODY'S NUTRITIONAL NEEDS AT THE DNA LEVEL

- Take the example of Daniel and the three Hebrew boys. Daniel and His three Hebrew friends were captives of the Babylonian king for the purpose of serving him in his palace. They were to be nourished and educated by the king for three years. Daniel and his friends purposed in their hearts not to defile themselves with the king's rich food of meats and wine. They asked for a test of ten days. During this time, they only drank water and ate pulse, which according to Josephus, consisted of sprouted beans, (Paulien 1997, p. 98). At the end of ten days they appeared fairer and fatter than all the other children that ate the king's rich food. They continued eating that way for the entire three years. At the end of that time they were tested and found to be ten times wiser and more intelligent than all the officials of the land (See Dan. 1).

- After ten days on this program, you will see wonderful effects, as well. Keep going to the end.
- Each cell's DNA is made up of minerals, amino acids (protein) and polysaccharides. This is the **MAP** for repairing and restoring your health.

MINERALS

Come from natural salts and vegetables (especially green, leafy vegetables).

NATURAL SALTS: Ocean Salt, Celtic salts, or Himalayan salt. Avoid regular refined sea salt and regular salt.

WHAT ABOUT SALT?

For humans, salt is as essential as water. We can perish from too little salt, just like we can from thirst. Salt regulates the exchange of water between our cells and their surrounding fluids. It is important for normal body functions. However, too much of the wrong kind of salt is bad for you. The right salt helps you stay hydrated, reduces fluid retention, provides a large amount of minerals, prevents muscle cramps, and nourishes the adrenal glands. "Sodium is the prominent element in body fluids. Our BLOOD, SWEAT, and TEARS are all salty like SEAWATER. The chemical composition of SEAWATER is virtually identical to that of HUMAN BLOOD. Hence, seawater contains all the minerals and trace elements necessary to build and sustain health" (Paulien 1997, p. 279).

Regular table salt and store brought sea salt is made up of 40% sodium and 60% chloride, with or without iodine.

Salt should be eaten the way it is found in nature. Nature's perfect balance will keep the body in perfect health. Disease will not grow in a healthy body.

The ocean water contains ninety-two minerals, and unprocessed salt from the ocean contains eighty minerals. (The rest are too minute to harvest.) Celtic salt and Himalayan salt have eighty to eighty-two minerals. The body needs these minerals for total healing.

The common salt found in the stores only has two to three minerals in unnatural proportions, which causes an imbalance in the body and brings about a host of diseases. IT HAS LOST ITS SAVOR (MINERALS) AND IS GOOD FOR NOTHING.

Natural sources of sodium are garlic, lemon, and celery.

NATURAL OCEAN SALTS will

- * Normalize BLOOD PRESSURE.
- * Regulate HEARTBEAT (stabilizes when drinking enough water).
- * Eliminate MUCUS BUILDUP (asthma, sinuses, and allergies).
- * Improve BRAIN function and remove toxins.
- * Help to BALANCE BLOOD SUGAR.
- * ALKALIZE the body by balancing the acid-alkaline affect.
- * Increase ENERGY on the cellular level.
- * Provide electrolyte balance by reducing WATER RETENTION (aid in weight loss).
- * Build IMMUNITY against disease.

* Help HEAL WOUNDS fast.
* CALM NERVES for restful SLEEP and prevents nighttime urination.
* Prevent muscle CRAMPS.

FRESH GREEN VEGETABLES: celery, cabbage, kale, turnip, brussels sprouts, broccoli, cauliflower, asparagus, beets, carrots, cucumbers, garlic, green and red peppers, lettuce (except iceberg), onions, potatoes, yams, spinach, sprouts, zucchini.

AMINO ACIDS (PROTEIN)

They come from legumes (beans), nuts, and seeds.

LEGUMES (BEANS): Lentils, kidney beans, soybeans, black eyed peas, green peas, black beans, garbanzos (chickpea), great northern beans, split peas, green or brown lentils, lima beans, navy beans, pinto beans, small red beans, soybeans.

NUTS (eat raw): Almonds, almond butter, brazil nuts, pecans, macadamia, cashews, hazel nuts, walnuts, brazil nuts, unsweetened coconut, flax seeds, peanuts, natural peanut butter.

Note: Some peanuts have mold and fat in them. Use natural peanut butter. Compare the labels of two jars: The one with the oil floating will only have peanuts and salt, and the one that has no oil on top will have additional ingredients.

SEEDS (eat raw): Pumpkin, sunflower, flaxseed, sesame, chia, and hemp.

YOUR CHALLENGES ARE:

__to eat a simple breakfast and dinner.

__to keep meals 6 hours apart. For example, space dinner/breakfast times as follows: 7 a.m. and 1 p.m. / or 8 a.m. and 2 p.m./ or 9 a.m. and 3 p.m.

BREAKFAST

Whole or sprouted grain (brown rice, quinoa, oatmeal, etc.)

* 2–3 kinds of fruit
* Nuts or seeds

LUNCH

Cooked whole or sprouted grain (brown rice, quinoa, etc.)

* A protein source (lentils, beans, nuts, tofu)
* Raw salad and steamed vegetables/greens
* Bread—whole/sprouted grain

SUPPER

* Fruit salad, a smoothie, soup, or popcorn. (Popcorn helps with acid reflux.) It is best to eat no supper because it is usually too close to bedtime. The last meal should be three to four hours before bed. "The sleep of such is generally disturbed with unpleasant dreams, and in the morning they awake unrefreshed. There is a sense of languor (lack of physical or mental energy) and loss of appetite. A lack of energy is felt through the entire system. In a short time the digestive organs are worn out, for they have had no time to rest" (White 1976, p. 174).

__to do a **SECOND MILE ACT** for someone:

__**to claim this promise:** *"…All thy waves and thy billows are gone over me. Yet the Lord will command his lovingkindness in the daytime, and in the night his song shall be with me, and his song shall be with me, and my prayer unto the God of my life"* (Ps. 42:7, 8).

RECIPES FOR THE DAY

A great dinner alternative

VEGETABLE BROTH:

3 medium carrots

3 medium Irish potatoes with skin

1 cup celery

1 medium onions, cut in half

3 garlic cloves

3 sprigs thyme or 1 tsp. powder thyme

3 quarts pure water

ADD water to all ingredients and simmer for 2 hours. Strain, and then add salt or homemade stock powder to taste.

STOCK POWDER

5 Tbsp. salt

1 ½ Tbsp. onion powder

2 Tbsp. garlic powder

2 Tbsp. sweet paprika

1 ½ Tbsp. oregano

5 Tbsp. dry parsley

1 ½ Tbsp. basil

¼ tsp. celery salt

1 tsp. turmeric

Season to taste.

CRACKERS

3 cup quick oats

2 cup unbleached flour

1 cup wheat germ

½ tsp. salt

¾ cup olive oil

1 cup water

MIX well. Roll thin on cookie sheet; score and bake at 325 degrees for 30 minutes.

MENTAL & MORAL AWARENESS

STEPS OF THE SANCTUARY PRAYER WALK

◆ At **His Altar of Intercession** while praying for others: Start with the Lord's Prayer and then get specific for friends, relatives, and enemies (1 Peter 2:5; Heb. 7:25). In the Old Testament, the fire was kindled by God Himself, and was sacredly cherished. Day and night, the holy incense diffused its fragranced throughout the sacred apartments, and far around the tabernacle (Ex. 37:26–28).

In the typical Old Testament service, the priest looked by faith to the mercy seat, which he could not see. The people of God are now to direct their prayers to Christ, their great High Priest, who, unseen by human vision, is pleading on their behalf in the sanctuary above.

The incense ascending with the prayers of Israel represents the merits and intercession of Christ. His perfect righteousness, through faith, is imputed to His people. This alone can make the worship of sinful beings acceptable to God.

WHAT DOES THE BIBLE SAY?

How to be Saved

- What question did the jailer ask *(Acts 16:30)*?
- What must we do to be saved *(John 3:16)*?
- How do we know God loves us *(Rom. 5:8)*?
- How do we become justified *(Rom. 3:23, 24)*?
- What else will God do for us *(John 1:12)*?

✓ *DAILY WELLNESS CHECK*

__*Did I eat more fruits and vegetables today?*

__*Was I intimate with God today?*

__*Am I ready for bed on time today?*

__*Did I drink enough water today?*

__*Did I overdo anything today?*

__*Did I exercise today?*

__*Am I taking deep breaths today?*

__*Did I get enough sunshine today?*

__*Did I dress appropriately today?*

MY PRAYERS & CHALLENGES

……

……

……

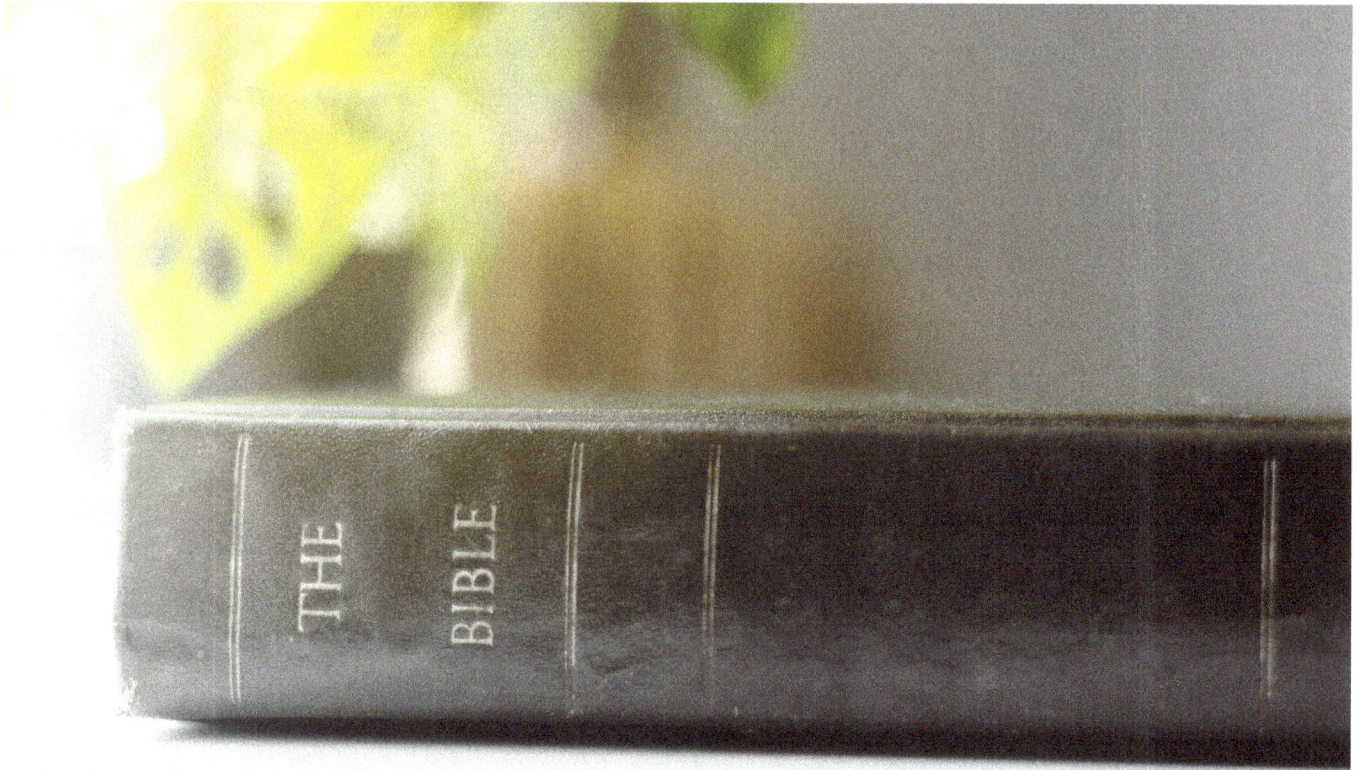

Physical Awareness

DEVELOPING THAT INTIMACY WITH GOD

HOW TO KNOW HIM PERSONALLY—To know Him is to love Him. We only get to know our Savior when we spend time with Him in the morning and the evening, and moment by moment throughout each day.

SPEND YOUR FIRST HOURS WITH HIM—Isaiah 50:4 says, "He wakeneth morning by morning, he wakeneth mine ear to hear as the learned. [as one who is taught]." When He wakes you in the morning at two, three, or four a.m., respond and start your worship right then. Christ followed that habit by waking up a great while before dawn to commune with His father. "And in the morning, rising up a great while before day, he went out, and departed into a solitary place, and there prayed" (Mark 1:35).

DEVELOPING FAITH—To develop your faith in God, read the Bible daily and make your requests known to Him. Ask, listen, and watch for answers to your prayers. Record your answers so that you can recount what He has done in the past. Your faith grows as you recount how God has worked for you. Your faith also grows as your awareness of the presence of God grows. Be aware that the angels are your constant companions, and that Christ and our Father are watching you. We should take notice that the enemy of our soul is watching also, but do not be afraid. He trembles when the weakest person prays to God the Father in the name of Jesus Christ, our Savior and Lord.

Jesus Christ (Yeshua), our Lord and Savior, is our only staying power. When a crisis comes, most of us will do everything else in the world to take care of the problem and leave Him as the last resort. But if we knew and loved Him like we know and love our earthly family and friends, we would call on Him first, instead of on others.

YOUR CHALLENGES ARE:

__to start and end worship with prayer.

__to sing several songs from your hymnal, or some you wrote yourself.

__to randomly open the Bible and read the first thing you set your heart on. Believe it and receive it as a promise, or an answer to a problem you are having.

__to pray (talk) sincerely as to a friend. Use the text that you read in your prayer. Be real when you are praying. Be humble and reverent.

__to do a **SECOND MILE ACT** for someone:

__**to claim this promise:** *"According to your faith be it unto you"* (Matt. 9:29).

RECIPE FOR THE DAY

CORNMEAL WAFFLES

3 cups water

2 cups corn meal

1 cup whole wheat flour

1 Tbsp. Rumford® baking powder (contains no aluminum)

2 Tbsp. honey

1 tsp. salt

¼ cup coconut oil

BLEND until smooth, then bake in your favorite waffle iron.

MENTAL & MORAL AWARENESS

A PRAYER FOR OTHERS

Father, I pray:

That their eyes would be opened.

That they would turn from darkness to light.

That they would turn from the power of Satan unto Elohiym (God).

That thy may receive forgiveness of sins and an inheritance with those who are sanctified (made holy) through faith in Yeshuah (Jesus) our Savior.

WHAT DOES THE BIBLE SAY?

How to Be Saved

- How is a man born again *(John 3:3–6)?*
- What does the born-again man do when tempted *(Rom. 6:16)?*
- Why should we keep God's law *(John 14:15)?*
- When Jesus comes, what will He do with our bodies *(Phil. 3:20,21)?*

✓ *DAILY WELLNESS CHECK*

__*Did I eat more fruits and vegetables today?*

__*Was I intimate with God today?*

__*Am I ready for bed on time today?*

__*Did I drink enough water today?*

__*Did I overdo anything today?*

__*Did I exercise today?*

__*Am I taking deep breaths today?*

__*Did I get enough sunshine today?*

__*Did I dress appropriately today?*

MY PRAYERS & CHALLENGES

....

....

....

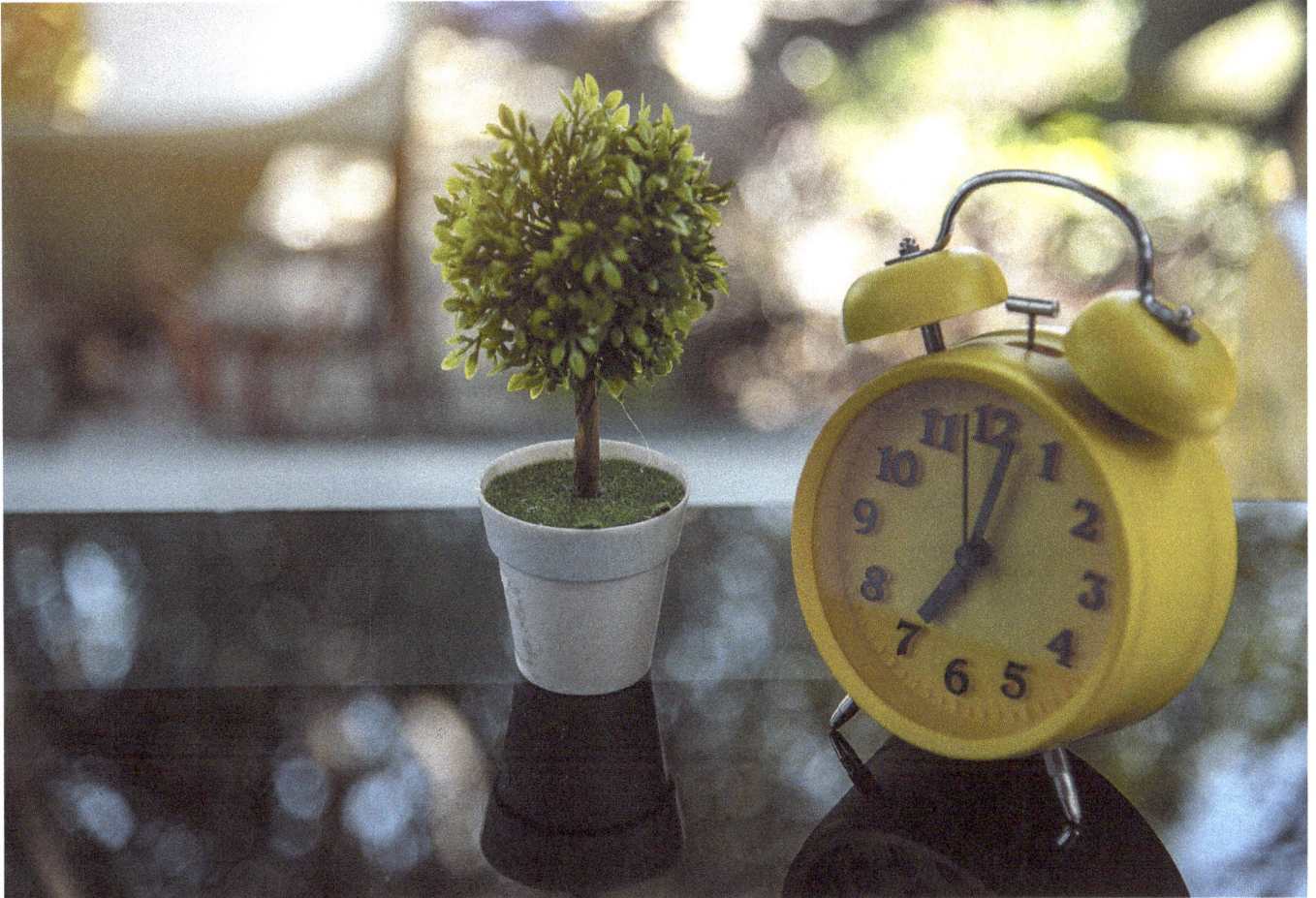

Physical Awareness

MORE FACTS ABOUT SLEEP

- To get the best rest, you must have regular sleeping hours.
- There is a built-in clock which is set by the regularity of sleeping hours and mealtimes.
- The best hours to sleep are the hours before midnight. Each hour before midnight makes the body feel like it has had two hours of sleep.
- A light supper, or no supper, will help.
- Your stomach should not be active while you are sleeping, therefore you should eat your last meal three to four hours before bedtime.
- A relaxing soak in warm water will help.
- You should sleep in a quiet, dark, well-ventilated room for the best rest.
- A little physical activity before retiring will improve rest.
- A clear conscience with the Lord and your fellow man will allow for excellent rest.

YOUR CHALLENGES ARE:

__to make sure there is no food in your stomach while you are sleeping.

__to keep lights off while sleeping.

__to take a nap before noon to slow down the aging process.

__to avoid stimulants like radio, television, tobacco, and caffeine.

__to avoid upsetting arguments, conversations, and confrontations in the evening.

__to set your worries and anxieties aside.

__to do a **SECOND MILE ACT** for someone:

__**to claim this promise:** *"He giveth power to the faint; and to them that have no might he increaseth strength"* (Isa. 40:29).

RECIPE FOR THE DAY

PANCAKES

2 cups water

2 cups whole wheat pastry flour

OR 1 cup of whole wheat flour with 1 cup of white flour

1 tsp. salt

2 Tbsp. Rumford baking powder (Try using Featherweight baking powder as a gluten free and sodium free option.)

2 Tbsp. honey

2 Tbsp. shredded coconut (optional)

BLEND until smooth. Spoon batter into a pan or onto a griddle at medium heat. Bake on each side until golden. Top with fruit spread.

MENTAL & MORAL AWARENESS

STEPS OF THE SANCTUARY PRAYER WALK

◆ Our final step in our prayer walk is into the **Most Holy Place.** You have now boldly come before the throne of grace to petition our Heavenly Father and Christ Our Lord and Savior for your daily needs and wants. Re-dedicate yourself here (Heb. 8:1, 2; 4:16). Wait patiently and listen silently for the Holy Spirit to speak to you. Do not be in a hurry to leave His Presence. Wait until you feel your prayer is heard.

WHAT DOES THE BIBLE SAY?

The Millennium

- What happens when the world ends *(John 14:1–3)*?
- Who will rise at the Second Coming *(1 Thess. 4:16, 17)*?
- Will the wicked ever be raised *(John 5:28, 29)*?
- What happens to the wicked at the Second Coming *(2 Thess. 1:7–9)*?
- How long will the righteous spend in heaven *(Rev. 20:4, 6)*?

✓ *DAILY WELLNESS CHECK*

__Did I eat more fruits and vegetables today?

__Was I intimate with God today?

__Am I ready for bed on time today?

__Did I drink enough water today?

__Did I overdo anything today?

__Did I exercise today?

__Am I taking deep breaths today?

__Did I get enough sunshine today?

__Did I dress appropriately today?

MY PRAYERS & CHALLENGES

………

………

………

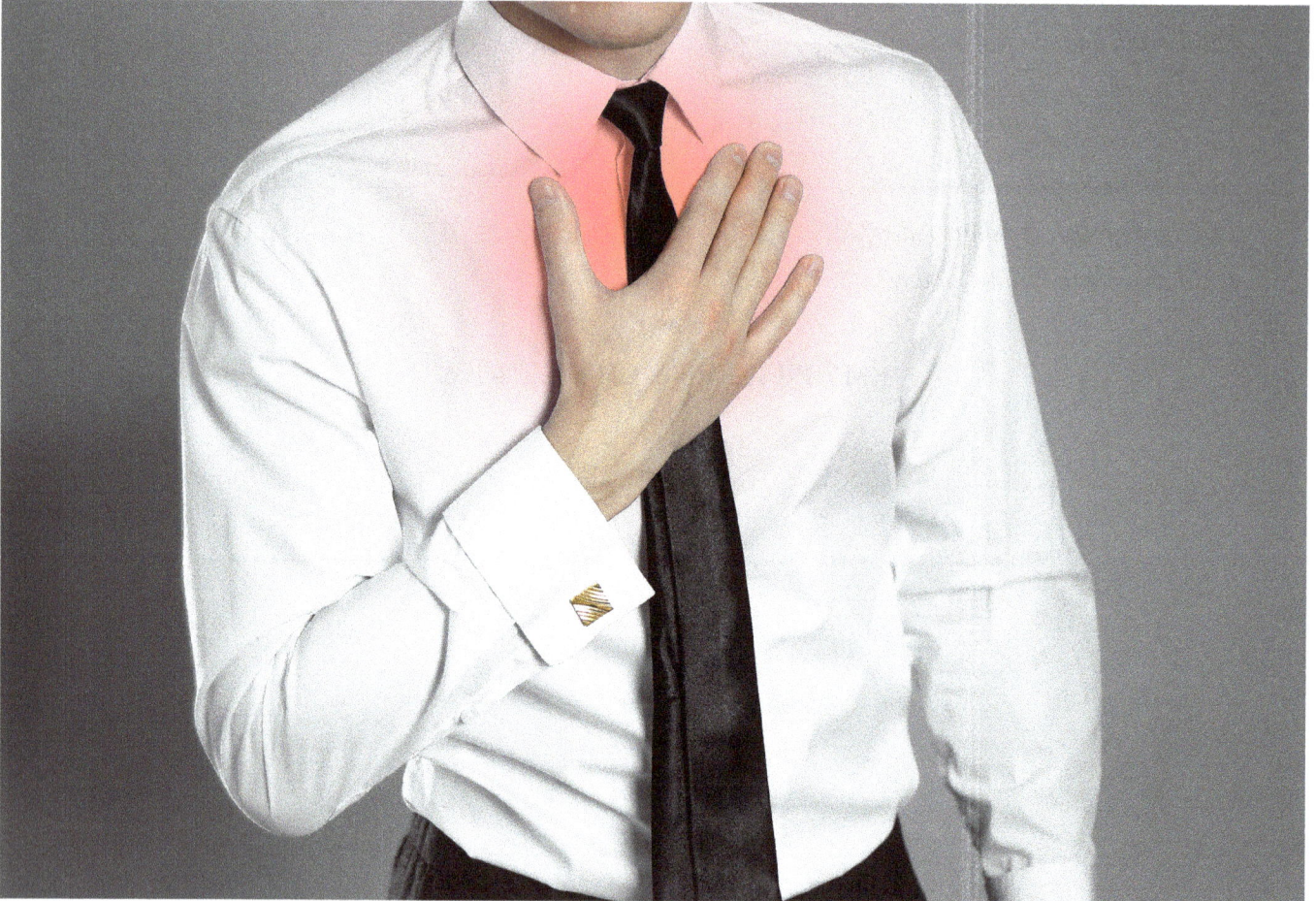

Physical Awareness

DRINK, DRINK, DRINK MORE WATER

Acid reflux! Acid reflux! Acid reflux!

Drinking with your meals is very detrimental to optimal health. The new so-called disease "acid reflux" or gastroesophageal reflux disease (GERD) is not a disease. It is an ailment created by several bad habits associated with eating.

When we drink cold drinks with meals, we must wait for two things to happen before our food can be digested. First, we must wait for the liquid to warm up to the same temperature as the stomach. Next, we must wait until all the liquid is absorbed. This slows down digestion and prolongs the time the food is in the stomach, creating an environment for fermentation and acid heartburn, or acid reflux. When we dilute the acid in the stomach, the weakened acid takes six to eight hours to digest the food, instead of the normal digestion time of three to four hours.

Another cause of acid reflux is eating or snacking between meals. For example, when you eat breakfast at 7 a.m., it will take the stomach four hours to digest all its contents. The stomach then needs one additional hour to rest before the next meal.

Instead you say, "I need a snack." So, you take your 10 a.m. break and have a snack. Your breakfast now has to stop digesting and wait for the snack to begin its digestion and come to the same consistency as the breakfast. Only then can the stomach complete its digestive process and empty its contents into the small intestines. This snack-digesting process will also take four hours. Only by two p.m. will the stomach finally be emptied.

But what about lunch? When you take your lunch at noon, the breakfast and the snack have to wait in the stomach until the noon meal gets to its consistency before all meals are emptied into the small intestines. If this cycle continues, other devastating diseases can occur besides just acid reflux.

YOUR CHALLENGES ARE:

__to avoid drinking with meals.

__to finish drinking water or liquids thirty minutes or more before a meal, and start drinking water again one to two hours after a meal. **Never drink liquids with your meals.** (If taking medication, no more than two to three ounces of water should be used to help take it.)

__to do a **SECOND MILE ACT** for someone:

__**to claim this promise:** *"Lord, I believe; help thou mine unbelief"* (Mark 9:24).

RECIPE FOR THE DAY

Peanut Butter and Banana Smoothie

2–3 ripe bananas

1–2 other fruits

1 cup of nut milk (coconut, rice, soy, or almond)

1 small spoon of natural peanut butter

¼ cup water (optional)

1 Tbsp. honey or maple syrup to taste

PEAL first and freeze very ripe bananas. Blend all ingredients until smooth.

MENTAL & MORAL AWARENESS

STEPS OF THE SANCTUARY PRAYER WALK

◆ In **His Most Holy Place,** which is beyond the veil, stands the center of the symbolic service of atonement and intercession, which forms the connecting link between heaven and earth (Rom. 5:11).

◆ **In this apartment was found the ark, a chest of acacia wood overlaid within and without with gold, and a crown of gold on the top (Ex. 25:11).**

◆ **The ark is where the tablet with the Ten Commandments, which God wrote Himself, lay. That is why it is also called the Ark of the Covenant, or the Ark of God's Testament (Ex. 34:28, 29; 25:21, 22).**

◆ **The Old Testament describes the ark as having Aaron's budded rod and a pot of manna. It was covered with the mercy seat, which was made of one solid piece of gold (Heb. 9:4).**

WHAT DOES THE BIBLE SAY?

The Millennium

- When will Satan be loosed from his prison *(Rev. 20:7)?*
- What will he do when set free *(Rev. 20:1, 3)?*
- When do the saints return to earth *(Rev. 21:1–3)?*
- When are the wicked dead resurrected *(Rev. 20:5)?*
- How does it all end *(Rev. 20:7–10)?*

✓ *DAILY WELLNESS CHECK*

__Did I eat more fruits and vegetables today?

__Was I intimate with God today?

__Am I ready for bed on time today?

__Did I drink enough water today?

__Did I overdo anything today?

__Did I exercise today?

__Am I taking deep breaths today?

__Did I get enough sunshine today?

__Did I dress appropriately today?

MY PRAYERS & CHALLENGES

……

……

……

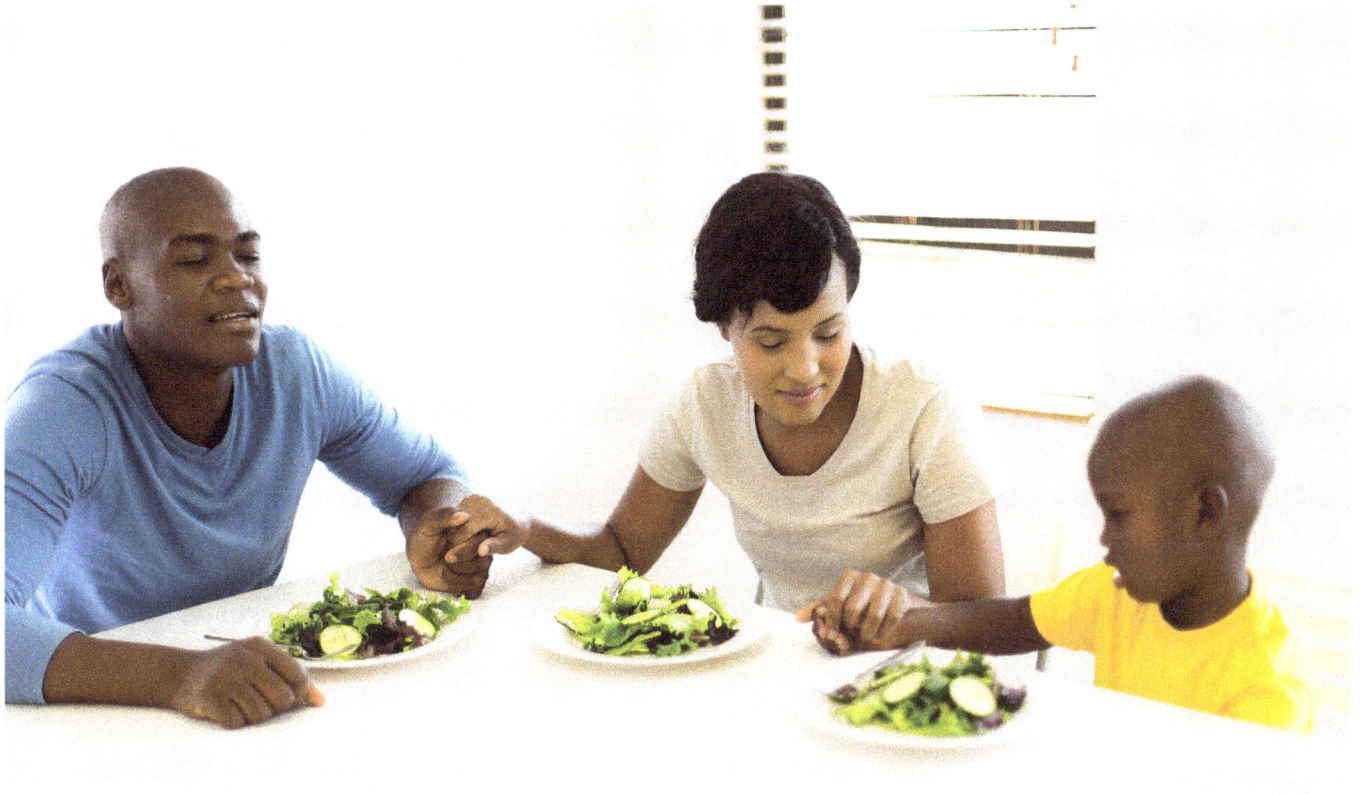

Physical Awareness

MORE ABOUT BEING CONSISTENLY TEMPERANT

The word "temperance," when used in the context of health, has three important meanings: moderation in the use of that which is good, total abstinence from that which is harmful, and self-restraint.

More is not always better. Working, exercising, resting, and eating are all needed, and beneficial to your health but if done to extreme, they can be harmful.

YOUR CHALLENGES ARE:

__to eat meals at the same time each day and wait five to six hours before the next meal starts.

__to avoid eating between meals.

__to use 1 tablespoon of **blackstrap molasses** with 1 tablespoon of lemon juice in a cup of hot water, instead of coffee, for energy and minerals.

__to do a **SECOND MILE ACT** for someone:

__**to claim this promise:** *"I can do all things through Christ which strengtheneth me"* (Phil. 4:13).

RECIPE FOR THE DAY

HUMMUS

1 cup garbanzo beans, canned or cooked

¼ cup hot water

2 Tbsp. tahini (optional, if you cannot find it; see below) **OR blend 1 cup sesame** (optional)

1 tsp. paprika

2 cloves minced garlic

½ tsp. cumin

2 Tbsp. lemon juice

1 tsp. salt

RINSE and drain garbanzo beans, then puree them with hot water in a blender. Last, blend in remaining ingredients until smooth, then serve. Consider adding some recommendations to dip in the hummus, like carrots, whole grain pita bread, etc.

OPTIONAL TAHINI RECIPE: If you cannot find Tahini or if wish to make your own from scratch: Toast in a frying pan 1 cup sesame seeds on medium heat until slightly brown. Transfer to a food processor or blender. Blend until smooth and pasty. Add 3 tablespoons grapeseed oil. Blend for 2-3 minutes, then add ½ teaspoon salt, blend again for 30 seconds and store in refrigerator. Tahini is a high source methionine, one of the twenty amino acids. This helps balance our hormones (Dence 2007, p. 85).

MENTAL & MORAL AWARENESS

Forgive Others

"And forgive us our debts, as we forgive our debtors. For if ye forgive men their trespasses, your heavenly Father will also forgive you: But if ye forgive not men their trespasses, neither will your Father forgive your trespasses" (Matt. 6:12, 14, 15).

Forgiveness means to excuse for a fault or offense, and to send the person you have forgiven away in peace.

Me Forgive *Them?*

If we require healing from the Lord, we must sincerely forgive those who hurt us. If this is not done, healing cannot fully take place. He who is not willing to forgive others, does not deserve to be forgiven. For God to extend forgiveness to an unforgiving person would be to approve that person's unforgiving spirit. To expect from others what one is unwilling to do himself, is the very essence of selfishness and sin. Only when we are right with our fellow man can we be made right with God. When we truly repent of our unforgiving spirit, God will free us from the debt of unforgiveness for the good of His perfect plan, and this is whether He chooses to heal us or not.

Here is a simple prayer: *Father, please give me love, joy, and peaceful thoughts towards _____ (name) and please give _____ (name) love, joy and peaceful thoughts towards me.*

My Current Health Assessment

1. Do you apologize easily? Yes/No
2. Do you have anger issues? Yes/No? If yes, why do you think that is?
3. Are you willing to forgive? Yes/No

YOUR CHALLENGES ARE:

__to ask God to give you love, joy and peaceful thoughts towards your enemy, and to give them the same for you.

__**to claim this promise:** *"If we confess our sins, he is faithful and just to forgive us our sins, and to cleanse us from all unrighteousness"* (1 John 1:9).

WHAT DOES THE BIBLE SAY?

The Law of God

- Without the law, what would we be unaware of *(Rom. 4:15)?*

- How permanent is God's law *(Luke 16:17)?*

- How long does the Psalmist say God's precepts will endure *(Ps. 111:7, 8)?*

- Is God's law good *(Rom. 7:12)?*

- What was Jesus' attitude towards the law *(Matt. 5:17–19)?*

✓ *DAILY WELLNESS CHECK*

__*Have I been forgiving today?*

__*Did I eat more fruits and vegetables today?*

__*Was I intimate with God today?*

__*Am I ready for bed on time today?*

__*Did I drink enough water today?*

__*Did I overdo anything today?*

__*Did I exercise today?*

__*Am I taking deep breaths today?*

__*Did I get enough sunshine today?*

__*Did I dress appropriately today?*

MY PRAYERS & CHALLENGES

....

....

....

A SAMPLE SANCTUARY PRAYER

Say what is in your *heart!*

Father, as I come into Your presence through Your gates, I praise you and thank you for_____.

At Your altar of sacrifice, I thank you for the merits of the blood of Christ that covers my sins. I repent and confess that I_____(sins).

Please cleanse me and renew my heart. Take away_____ (old habits and attitudes). Wash me at the laver of washing.

Now that I am washed, Father, please clothe me with Christ's robe of righteousness. I have faith in His righteous, that you will give me strength to do all things you ask of me.

Bless me with Your faith, virtue, knowledge, temperance, patience, godliness, brotherly kindness, and love. Give me the love that is found in 1 Corinthians 13:4–8. (Repeat once.)

Father, as I raise my hands so You can symbolically put Your Son's robe of righteousness on me. Please also place your armor on me; piece by piece. I also need You to guard the avenues to my soul: my eyes, my ears, my nose, my taste (mouth), and my hands (touch).

I now enter into Your Holy Place. I am at the lampstand of the Holy Spirit. I ask again today for the baptism of Your Holy Spirit. I open my mouth wide so You can fill it, as You said in Psalms 81:10, "Open thy mouth wide, and I will fill it," and as stated in Job 29:23, "And they waited for me as for the rain; and they opened their mouth wide as for the latter rain."

I need the Spirit of wisdom, understanding, knowledge, discernment, counsel, fear of God, and power. I also need the **fruit of Your Spirit** *(Repeat them from Galatians 5:22)* for myself, and love, joy, and peace towards those who are not at peace with me. Give them the same love, joy, and peace towards me.

I am now at the **table of shew bread, or the table of His presence,** which represents Your Word. Today, You shared with me_____ (Bible or other special reading), and I am meditating on them. They are exactly what I needed today. Please help me to _____.

I am now at Your **alter of intercession,** where I will pray for my family, friends, and others.

I am now in the **Most Holy Place,** mentally. I enjoy the warm companionship of Christ as He walks with me through the Sanctuary. I love you, my heavenly Father, and Yeshua, my Savior. Thank you for providing _____ for me. I **need_____ and want _____**, if it is Your will. I **rededicate** myself to YOU.

Wait patiently and listen silently for His responses.

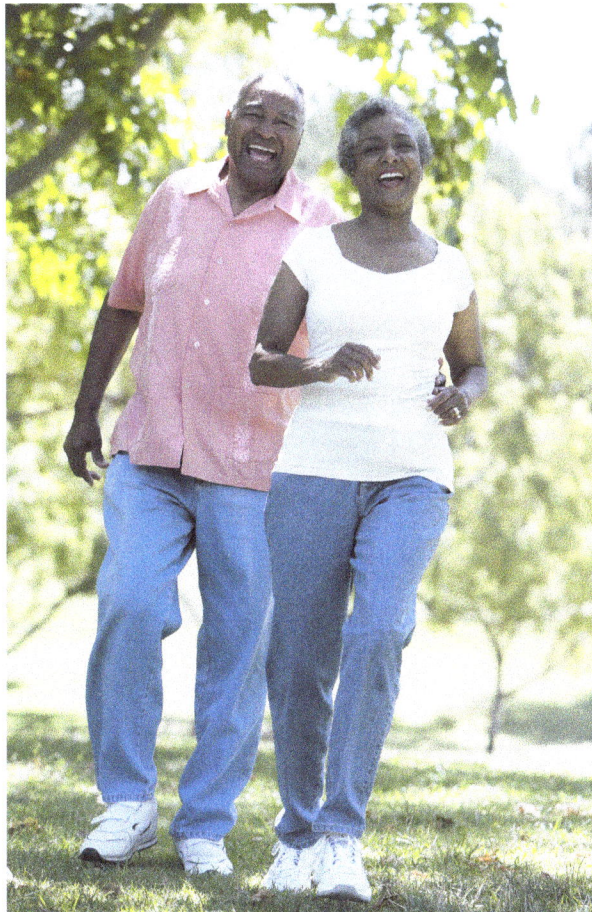

Physical Awareness

MORE FACTS ABOUT EXERCISING DAILY

A good workout forces you to breathe deeply and speeds up the circulation of oxygen-rich blood throughout the body. It helps you feel good and is affective in fighting off depression, stress, and anxiety.

Walking is best because it uses almost all 206 bones and 640 muscles that we have. It is easy on your joints, and you can walk at your own pace.

YOUR CHALLENGES ARE:

__to spend more time outdoors. It will help give you a positive attitude. Perform aerobic exercise in the fresh air every other day.

__to lift weights or do sit-ups on the other days. (These are called resistance exercises.)

__to try the **burst training technique:** Run in place as fast as you possibly can for 15 seconds, rest for 45 seconds, do it again for a total of 7 times. Exercising for 7 minutes will **burn fat for 48 hours.** You can increase the time to 30 seconds, and the rest time for 1.5 minutes. Do this workout every other day.

NOTE: Stop if it hurts! Exercise to the intensity that you are barely able to carry on a conversation as you exercise. If you develop chest pains during exercise, stop at that point. When you have reached the point in exercise where you are barely able to carry on a conversation, take your pulse.

How to take your 10-seconds pulse rate:

Place your index and middle fingers on your wrist, palm up on the side with your thumb, and count the number of beats for ten seconds. Multiply the number of beats you counted by six, and you will know your one-minute pulse rate.

How to relieve pain and remove toxins:

__Take 2–3 cabbage leaves and bruise them with a hammer, a bottle, or a rolling pin. Place on the aching or swollen part and wrap it to yourself with a compressive device, like Ace® bandage, plastic cling, or kerlix.

OR

__Rub area with a mixture of 8 ounces of cold pressed peanut oil, and the juice from 5–6 freshly squeezed and strained lemons.

OR

__Rub the area with avocado oil; it has incredible healing properties. If inflamed, rub the area with tea tree or eucalyptus oil.

__to do a **SECOND MILE ACT** for someone:

__**to claim this promise:** "*…Lo, I am with you alway, even unto the end of the world. Amen*" (Matt. 28:20).

RECIPES FOR THE DAY

ALMOND MILK

1 cup water

½ tsp. honey

½ cup raw almonds

¼ tsp. natural almond flavoring (opt.)

½ tsp. vanilla extract

¼ tsp. salt

4 cups water

SOAK almonds in hot water for 10 minutes. Pull skin off of almond and use only the white of the almonds. Blend first 6 ingredients on high for 1–2 minutes or until creamy. Then, add 4 cups of water. Blend briefly. Chill.

GREEN SMOOTHIE

2 cups kale

1 cup spinach

5 stems parsley

½ cup pineapple (canned, fresh, or frozen)

2 Tbsp. lecithin

1 Tbsp. flax seeds

1 Tbsp. chia seeds

BLEND all ingredients with pineapple juice. You can half all of the ingredient amounts for a smaller serving size.

GREEN LEAFY BLEND

For a smoothie focused on getting the chlorophyll and minerals that you need:

Blend 1 cup of any 4 green, leafy vegetables for 1 minute in 8 ounces of water; strain and drink 4–6 ounces.

MENTAL & MORAL AWARENESS

Offer a Praise and Thanksgiving

"Be careful for nothing; but in every thing by prayer and supplication with thanksgiving let your requests be made known unto God" (Phil. 4:6).

"And whatsoever ye do in word or deed, do all in the name of the Lord Jesus, giving thanks to God and the Father by him" (Col. 3:17).

FACTS ABOUT HOW TO OFFER PRAISE AND THANKSGIVING

- Have a spirit of gratitude and praise, and resist a spirit of melancholy, discontented thoughts, and feelings.
- Your mind is clouded when you are in pain; therefore do not try to overthink during these times. You know that Jesus loves you. He understands your weakness. When you feel overwhelmed, you may do His will by simply resting in His arms.
- It is a law of nature that our thoughts and feelings are encouraged and strengthened when expressed (White 2001, 419.3). Therefore, you need to express your faith by rejoicing more in the blessings that you know you have, which included the great mercy and love of God.
- No tongue can express, no finite mind can conceive, the blessings that result from appreciating the goodness and love of God. Even on earth, we may have joy as a wellspring which never fails, because we are fed by the stream that flows from the throne of God.
- Never forget that we must abide in the light shining from the cross of Calvary, and that we are children of the heavenly King. We are sons and daughters of the Lord of Hosts. It is our privilege to rest calmly in God.

"And let the peace of God rule in your hearts ... and be ye thankful" (Col. 3:15).

My Current Health Assessment

1. Is it easy for you to say "thank you"? Yes/No
2. Are you angry with unthankful people? Yes/No
3. Do you attribute it to God when good thinks happen to you? Yes/No

THE CHALLENGE IS:

__to give thanks at all times, and for all things.

__to look around you and see all the things you are thankful for.

WHAT DOES THE BIBLE SAY?

The Law of God

Can we throw away any part of the law *(James 2:10)?*

How many commandments are found in the New Testament *(Matt. 22:36–40)?*

What does it mean to love God *(1 John 5:1–3)?*

How does God know that we love Him? *(1 John 2:3–6)?*

How are God's last-day people identified *(Rev. 14:12)?*

✓ *DAILY WELLNESS CHECK*

__*Am I still forgiving today?*

__*Am I being thankful today?*

__*Did I eat more fruits and vegetables today?*

__*Was I intimate with God today?*

__*Am I ready for bed on time today?*

__*Did I drink enough water today?*

__*Did I overdo anything today?*

__*Did I exercise today?*

__*Am I taking deep breaths today?*

__*Did I get enough sunshine today?*

__*Did I dress appropriately today?*

MY PRAYERS & CHALLENGES

....

....

....

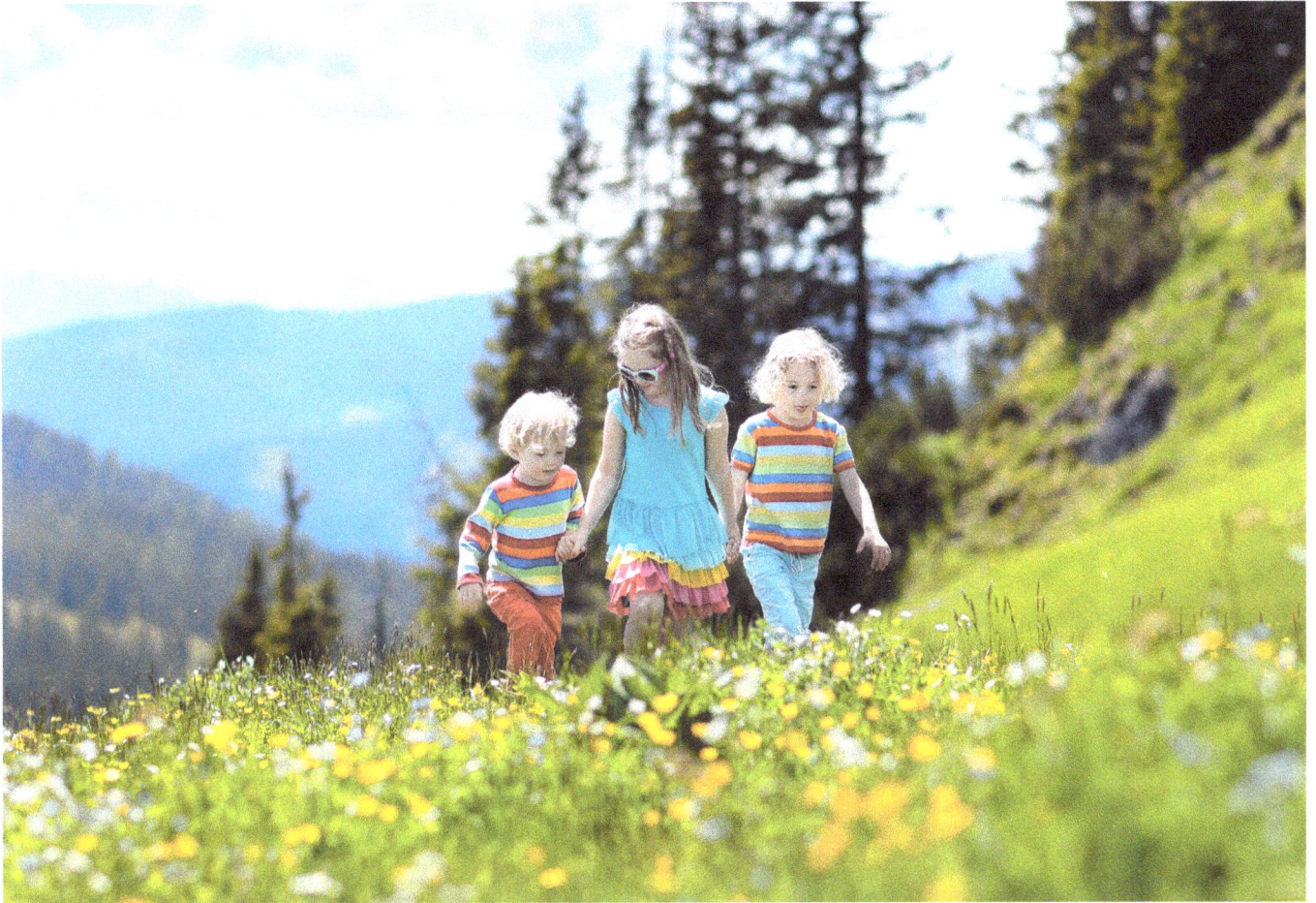

Physical Awareness

MORE FACTS ABOUT PURE, FRESH AIR

- It stimulates the appetite and helps the food to digest more perfectly.
- It promotes healthful circulation of the blood.
- It refreshes and strengthens the body.
- It soothes the nerves and gives the mind composure and serenity.
- Every cell must receive a constant supply of air to strengthen it. Without air, the cells will die and so will you.
- Mankind and animals take in oxygen from the air and give off carbon dioxide, while plants use the carbon dioxide and give off oxygen. Nature balances itself.

- For the best rest, keep a window slightly open while sleeping, but not directly on you. Wear cotton or natural fiber sleepwear to bed because they breathe better on the skin. Headaches can be caused by breathing stale or polluted air.

YOUR CHALLENGES ARE:

__to stand erect.

__to sit as if you are a puppet, like a string is attached to your chest and being pulled up towards the ceiling.

__to do a **SECOND MILE ACT** for someone:

__**to claim this promise:** *"Delight thyself also in the Lord; and he shall give thee the desires of thine heart"* (Ps. 37:4).

RECIPE FOR THE DAY

CORN BREAD or MUFFINS

1½ cups cornmeal

1½ cups wheat pastry flour

1 tsp. sea salt

1½ Tbsp. baking powder

¼ cup coconut milk (optional)

3 Tbsp. honey

2 cups water

PREHEAT oven to 350 degrees. Mix all dry ingredients together in one bowl and spoon into muffin pan. Bake in greased pan for 30 minutes.

MENTAL & MORAL AWARENESS

Love Life

"A merry heart doeth good like a medicine: but a broken spirit drieth the bones" (Prov. 17:22).

Loving life is extremely essential to your wellbeing. When we do not love life, we act out destructive behaviors towards ourselves and others. The Word of God is life, and to know God is to love Him. Therefore, to love life adds up to knowing God through His word, the Bible.

FACTS ABOUT HOW TO LOVE LIFE

- Reading the word of God every day and meditating on it, brings life into your being.
- Doing good for others will make you feel good all over.
- "Rejoice in the Lord always: and again I say, Rejoice" (Phil. 4:4). If you cannot rejoice, ask for a merry heart, just as you would ask for all the other things that you want.

My Current Health Assessment:

1. Are you happy every morning? Yes/No/Sometimes

2. Are most of your friends positive people? Yes/No

3. Do you remain positive when discouraging things happen? Yes/No/Sometimes

YOUR CHALLENGES ARE:

__to think positive thoughts.

__to speak positive words.

__to keep positive friends around you.

__to ask your Father in heaven to send you positive associates.

WHAT DOES THE BIBLE SAY?

The Sabbath

- What did God do after creating the world (*Gen 2:1-3*)?
- Did God mention the Sabbath in His commandments (*Ex. 20:8–11*)?
- Of what is the Sabbath a sign (*Ezek. 20:12, 20*)?
- What blessing comes to those who keep the Sabbath (*Isa. 58:12–14*)?
- Did Jesus worship on the Sabbath (*Luke 4:16*)?

✓ *DAILY WELLNESS CHECK*

__*Am I still forgiving today?*

__*Am I being thankful today?*

__*Am I happy today?*

__*Did I eat more fruits and vegetables today?*

__*Was I intimate with God today?*

__*Am I ready for bed on time today?*

__*Did I drink enough water today?*

__*Did I overdo anything today?*

__*Did I exercise today?*

__*Am I taking deep breaths today?*

__*Did I get enough sunshine today?*

__*Did I dress appropriately today?*

MY PRAYERS & CHALLENGES

....

....

....

HEALTHY TIDBITS

Things that slow down metabolism

- Stress
- Alcohol
- Overeating
- Snacking
- Large amount of fluid with meals

Things that speed up the metabolism

- Exercise
- Get an adequate amount of sleep. Research shows that sleep deprivation and sleep disorders may have profound metabolic and cardiovascular implication (Sharma 2010).
- Take two tablespoons lemon juice before or after meals

Hormones are increased with:

- Laughter
- Exercise
- Sunshine
- Sleeping in the dark
- Fasting in the morning

Hormones are decreased with:

- Worry
- Artificial light
- Caffeine
- Alcohol
- Meat

RECIPE FOR THE DAY

NATURAL IRON DRINK

1 cup blackstrap molasses

1 cup figs

1 cup prunes

1 cup raisins

1 cup apricots

1 gal grape juice

LET this sit for 24 hours. Drink 4 ounces 2 times a day.

A HIGH BLOOD PRESSURE CONTROL

Besides drinking 2 to 3 quarts of water daily: Take one clove of garlic and press it flat. Place it in a cup for 10 minutes; then, pour hot water into a cup and cover for an additional 10 minutes. After this, you can put in a pinch of cayenne pepper, and sip on the beverage. Drinking 1 to 2 cups a day will help naturally control blood pressure.

WARNING: If you are taking blood thinners, limit how much garlic you intake. CHOOSE PRAYFULLY and consult your pharmacist or doctor about possible drug interactions

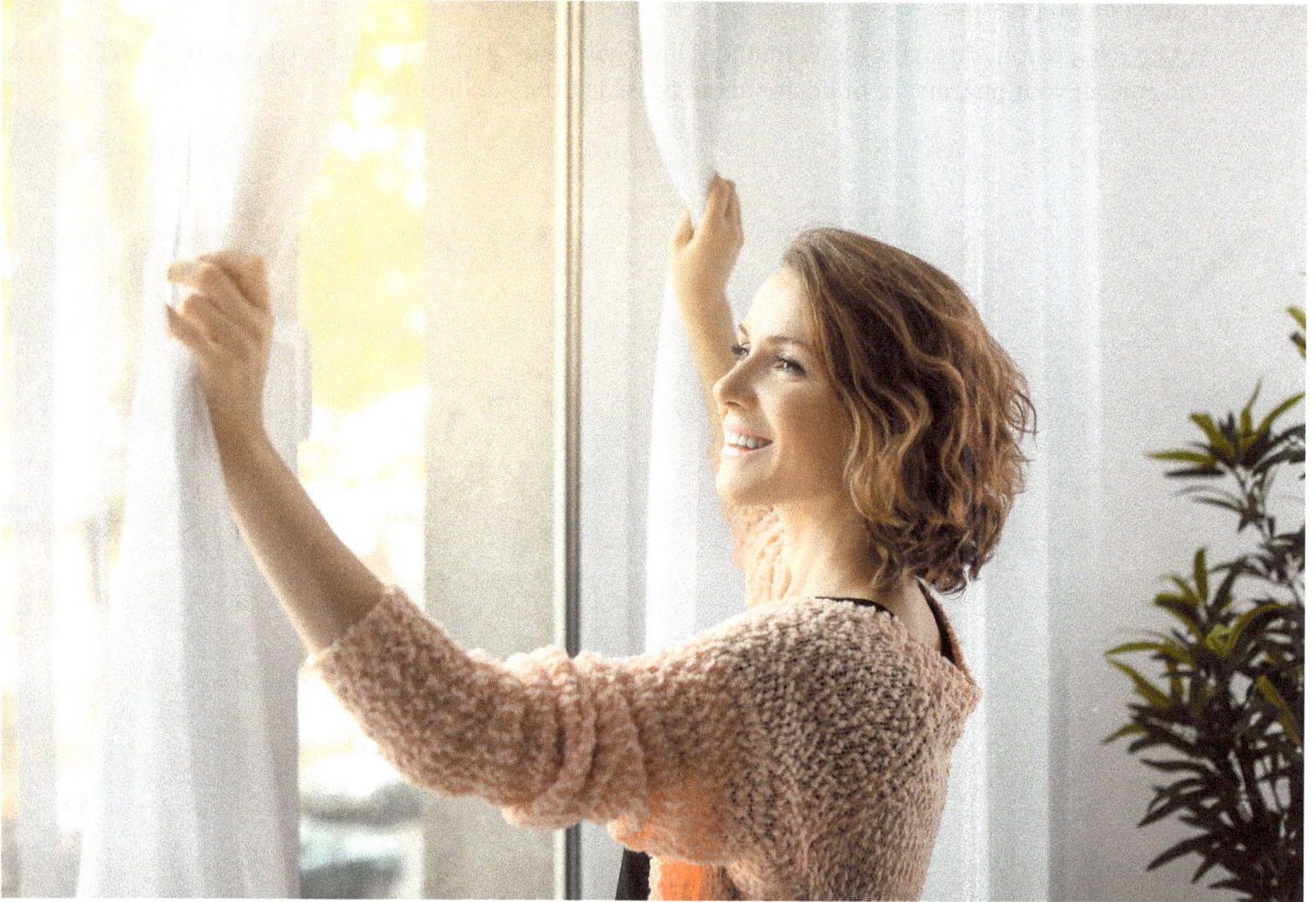

Physical Awareness

FACTS ABOUT WHY TO KEEP LETTING THE SUNLIGHT SHINE IN:

- Humans, like plants, need adequate sunlight.
- It helps to relax tension while enhancing your mental outlook and sense of well-being, because sunlight increases endorphins.
- It produces mental alertness and helps prevent or overcome mental depression.

YOUR CHALLENGES ARE:

__to be in the sunshine at least thirty minutes every day if you have darker skin.

__to be in the sunshine at least fifteen minutes every day if you have lighter skin.

__to do a **SECOND MILE ACT** for someone:

__**Claim This Promise:** *"Draw nigh to God, and he will draw nigh to you. Cleanse your hands…and purify your hearts …. Humble yourselves in the sight of the Lord, and he shall lift you up"* (James 4:8–10).

RECIPE FOR THE DAY

FRESH FRUIT or DRIED FRUIT JAM

1¼ cups dried fruit (chopped)

1 cup water or fruit juice

¼ cup arrowroot or corn starch

LIGHTLY boil the ingredients in a covered saucepan for 5–10 minutes or until the fruit is softened. MASH the spread with a fork to make a chunky spread or blend for a smooth spread.

MENTAL & MORAL AWARENESS

Lending a Helping Hand

"…*Then shall thy light break forth as the morning, and thine health shall spring forth speedily"* (Isa. 58:8).

Is this not the fast that I have chosen? to loose the bands of wickedness, to undo the heavy burdens, and to let the oppressed go free, that ye break every yoke? Is it not to deal thy bread to the hungry, and that thou bring the poor that are cast out to thy house? when thou seest the naked, that thou cover him; and that thou hide not thyself from thine own flesh? Then shall thy light break forth as the morning, and thy health shall spring forth speedily: and thy righteousness shall go before thee... (Isa. 58: 6–8; see Isa. 9–11).

FACTS ABOUT LENDING A HELPING HAND…

- One of the main things that slows down or stops your recovery, is to focus your attention on yourself. Many sick individuals feel that everyone should give them sympathy and help, when what they need is to have their attention turned away from themselves and towards caring for others.
- God answers prayer for those who place themselves in the channel of His blessings, by doing for others while they are sick.
- As we seek to comfort others with the same comfort we would want, the blessing comes back to us.

My Current Health Assessment:

1. Did you like doing your chores or running errands when you were young? Yes/No
2. Do you need others to do errands for you? Yes/No
3. How quickly do you do agree to perform errands for others? __Always __Sometimes __Never

YOUR CHALLENGES ARE:

__to watch for opportunities to help.

__to not put off a call, a prayer, a visit, or a good deed.

WHAT DOES THE BIBLE SAY?

The Sabbath

- What day did Paul keep *(Acts 17:2)?*
- How did the early believers keep the Sabbath *(Acts 13:42–44)?*
- Will the Sabbath be kept in heaven *(Isa. 66:22, 23)?*
- What day is called "the Lord's Day" *(Mark 2:27, 28)?*

✓ *DAILY WELLNESS CHECK*

__*Am I still forgiving today?*

__*Am I being thankful today?*

__*Am I happy today?*

__*Am I helpful today?*

__*Did I eat more fruits and vegetables today?*

__*Was I intimate with God today?*

__*Am I ready for bed on time today?*

__*Did I drink enough water today?*

__*Did I overdo anything today?*

__*Did I exercise today?*

__*Am I taking deep breaths today?*

__*Did I get enough sunshine today?*

__*Did I dress appropriately today?*

MY PRAYERS & CHALLENGES

....

....

....

HEALTHY TIDBITS

Advantages of Exercise and Recreation in the Form of Useful Labor

Work is a part of general conditioning for the body. Work helps you keep the appetites under control. Work brings into play all the muscles of the body and teaches judgement, mental resourcefulness and decision-making. It brings relief from taxing mental labor by the performance of repetitious physical acts.

We believe that the Lord specially blesses those who use mind and muscle in a practical way. We encourage you to engage freely in the volunteering of your time, energy, and strength in doing useful labor. God's plan for the maintenance of the body equipment includes purposeful labor, not mere calisthenics.

Adam's exercise was appointed in the Garden of Eden and included purposeful labor. Work with the hands should never be considered degrading to one's position. Adam was the only man who has ever been considered the sole heir of the entire earth, yet he was a farmer who got his exercise in the garden.

Benefits of Work in Childhood

If you have children, their happiness is assured if they are taught to labor with their hands. Even though they may not like it during their early years, if they are taught how to do it, they will look to this as a means of recreation as they get older. Since it brings with it the blessings of the provisions for one's needs, it turns out to be a double blessing.

Another Quick Note for the Youth

Many of the youth are suffering from anxiety. Sounds crazy, right? Anxiety means they feel worried and uneasy. They are also intensely fearful of the future. These are your children, so you can help them start their own personal relationship with our Father, their Father in heaven. Encourage them to start with fifteen minutes at a time. They will learn to increase it themselves.

Please do this for them. It is important for your future, and for their futures.

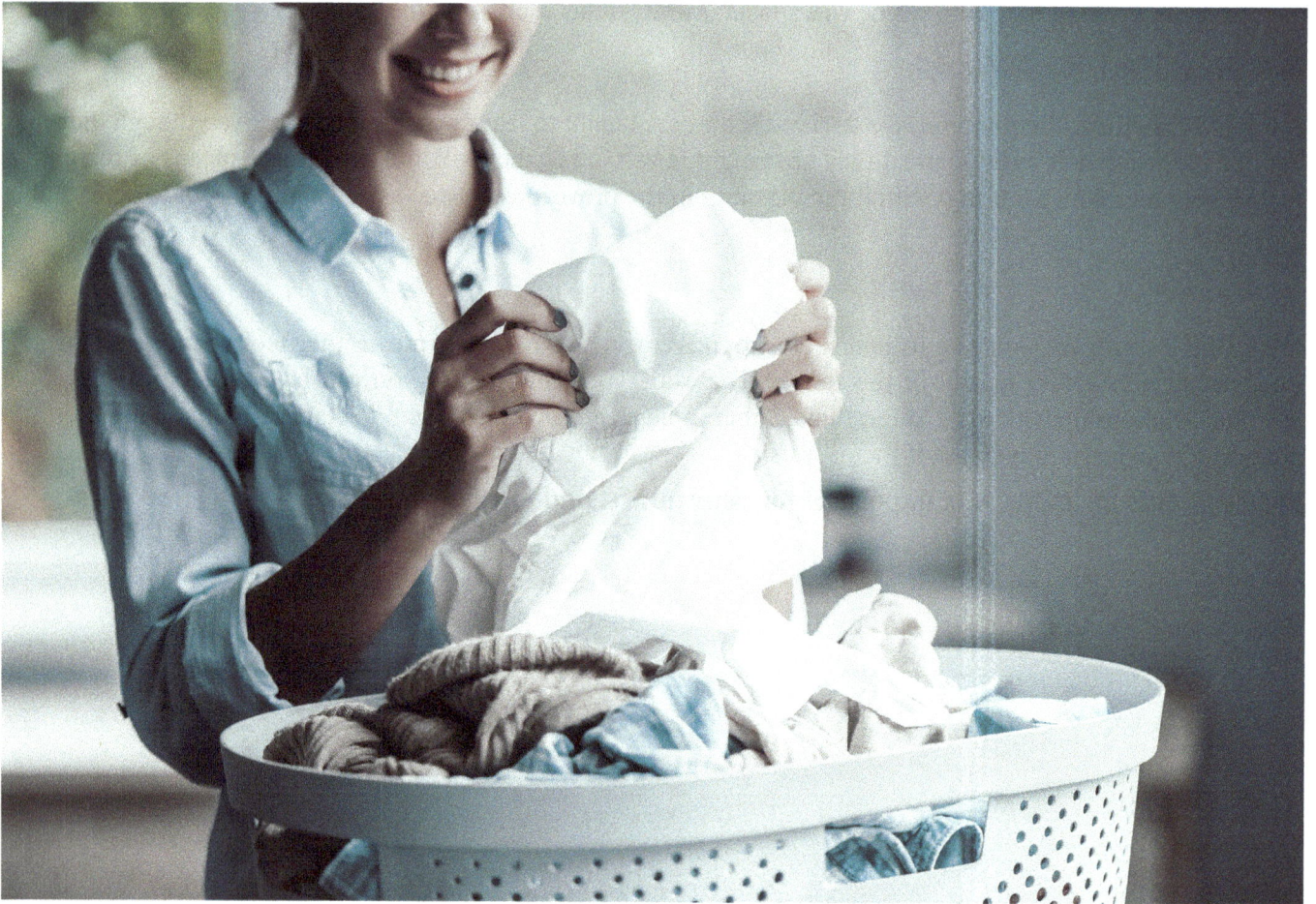

Physical Awareness

MORE FACTS ABOUT WEARING CLOTHES THAT PROMOTE HEALTH

- It is impossible to have the best of health if the extremities are habitually cold. The unequal circulation which results from clothing the trunk more warmly than the extremities, allows toxic materials to build up both in the anemic extremities and in the congested viscera. Blood tends to pool in any area of inflammation. In the head the excess blood produces headaches; I the chest it produces coughs, in the intestinal tract various types of discomfort, and in the kidneys inefficient cleaning of the blood. (Thrash 2013)

- Our clothing should be washed clean. Uncleanliness in dress is unhealthful and is defiling to the body and soul. "Ye are the temple of God.... If any man defile the temple of God, him shall God destroy" (1 Cor. 3:16, 17).

- In all respects, dress should be chosen to promote health. God desires us to be in health of both body and soul: "Beloved, I wish thee above all things that thou mayest prosper and be in health, even as thy soul prospereth" (3 John 2).

YOUR CHALLENGES ARE:

__to spring clean your closet.

__to do a **SECOND MILE ACT** for someone:

__**to claim this promise:** *"The Lord is at hand. Be careful for nothing; but in everything by prayer and supplication with thanksgiving let your requests be made known to God" (Phil 4:5, 6).*

RECIPE FOR THE DAY

MOM'S NATURAL FOOD ANTIBIOTIC

2 medium or 1 large onion (sliced)

3-4 Tbsp. garlic (crushed)

2-3 inches ginger root (grated)

1 Tbsp. Italian seasoning

COVER and boil for twenty minutes in one and a half quarts of water. My 81 year old mom drinks a cup every other night. She said it keeps her cleansed and rejuvenated and living with no illnesses or medications.

MENTAL & MORAL AWARENESS

Obey Willingly

"A blessing, if ye obey the commandments of the Lord your God, which I command you this day: And a curse, if ye will not obey the commandments of the LORD your God" (Deut. 11:27, 28).

The result of obedience to God's requirements brings the obedient person under the laws which control the physical being. Those who want to preserve their lives in health must prayerfully bring all their mental, spiritual, and physical appetites and passions, under the control of God.

Me, Obey Him?

Health, life, and happiness are the result of obedience to physical laws governing our bodies. If our will and way are in accordance with God's will and way, and if we do the pleasure of our Creator, He will keep the human organism in good condition. He will restore our moral, mental, and physical powers in order that He may work through us to His glory. His restoring power is constantly being manifested in our bodies. If we cooperate with Him, health and happiness, peace and usefulness, are the sure results.

My Current Health Assessment:

1. Were you an obedient child? Yes/No/Sometimes

2. Can you recognize when God is speaking to you? Yes/No/Sometimes

3. Are you aware that you are a child of God and that you owe Him obedience? Yes/No

THE CHALLENGE IS:

__to watch, pray, and listen for the voice of God in nature, the Bible, and in Providence.

WHAT DOES THE BIBLE SAY?

First Day of the Week

- What happened on the first day of the week *(Matt. 28:1)?*
- Read Mark's account *(Mark 16:2)*.
- Read Luke's account *(Luke 24:1)*.
- Read John's account *(John 20:1)*.

✓ *DAILY WELLNESS CHECK*

__*Am I still forgiving today?*

__*Am I being thankful today?*

__*Am I happy today?*

__*Am I helpful today?*

__*Am I obedient today?*

__*Did I eat more fruits and vegetables today?*

__*Was I intimate with God today?*

__*Am I ready for bed on time today?*

__*Did I drink enough water today?*

__*Did I overdo anything today?*

__*Did I exercise today?*

__*Am I taking deep breaths today?*

__*Did I get enough sunshine today?*

__*Did I dress appropriately today?*

MY PRAYERS & CHALLENGES

....

....

....

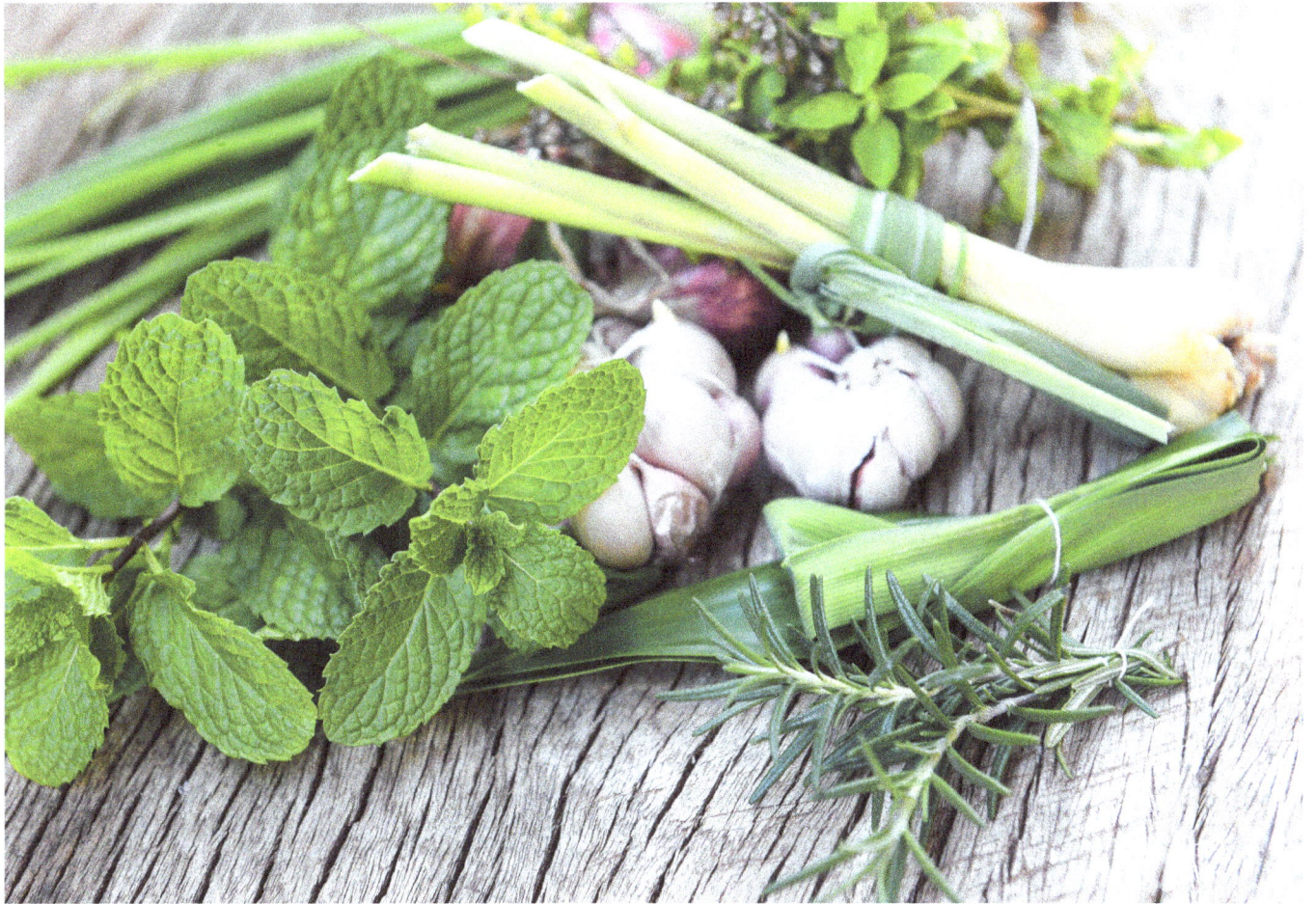

Physical Awareness

HERBS AND HOW TO USE THEM IN COOKING (Hurd, Frank and Hurd, Rosalie. "A Good Cook...TEN TALENTS" 1968, pp. 164-166)

CORIANDER (Ground fine)—Cinnamon substitute, apple pie, pumpkin pie, bread, waffles, cookies, cakes, cherry pudding

CUMIN—Stews, chili, kidney beans

DILL—Potato salad, pickling, gravy, sauerkraut, soups, tea-dill, cabbage-slaw

FENNEL FRONDS (tops)—Soups, lentils, beans, brown rice, tomato sauces (Can be chewed and are pleasant to taste)

FENNEL SEEDS—Herb teas, cookies, cakes, bread

GARLIC BULB—Soups, sauces, tomatoes, legumes, bread, crackers, baked potatoes, all salads

MARJORAM—Soups, stews, salads dressing, spaghetti sauces, vegetables, meatless roast

YOUR CHALLENGES ARE:

__to try using several new spices in your cooking.

__to do a **SECOND MILE ACT** for someone:

__**to claim this promise:** *"Because he hath set his love upon me, therefore will I deliver him: I will set him on high because he hath known my name"* (Ps. 91:14).

MENTAL & MORAL AWARENESS

To those who make the Savior's principles their guide, how precious are His words of promise:

"And why take ye thought for raiment? ... If God so clothe the grass of the field, which to day is, and to morrow is cast into the oven, shall he not much more clothe you? ... Therefore take no thought, saying, 'Wherewithal shall we be clothed?' ... For your heavenly Father knoweth that ye have need of all these things. But seek ye first the kingdom of God, and His righteousness; and all these things shall be added unto you" (Matt. 6:28, 30–33).

WHAT DOES THE BIBLE SAY?

First Day of the Week

- What did the disciples do on the first day *(Acts 20:7)?*
- What did Paul ask the Corinthian believers to do *(1 Cor. 16:2)?*
- What day did John have his vision on *(Rev. 1:10)?*
- Who was the Sabbath made for *(Mark 2:27, 28)?*

✓ *DAILY WELLNESS CHECK*

__*Am I still forgiving today?*

__*Am I being thankful today?*

__*Am I happy today?*

__*Am I helpful today?*

__*Am I obedient today?*

__*Did I eat more fruits and vegetables today?*

__*Was I intimate with God today?*

__*Am I ready for bed on time today?*

__*Did I drink enough water today?*

__*Did I overdo anything today?*

__*Did I exercise today?*

__*Am I taking deep breaths today?*

__*Did I get enough sunshine today?*

__*Did I dress appropriately today?*

MY PRAYERS & CHALLENGES

………

………

………

HEALTHY TIDBITS

Eating between meals

X-ray studies have been conducted to determine the emptying time of a normal stomach. Anything remaining in the stomach five hours after a test meal is abnormal. The stomach usually empties itself in 2 ½ to 4 hours. Series of tests have been run in which people have been given routine breakfasts consisting of cereal and cream, bread, cooked fruit, and an egg. These stomachs were x-rayed and found to be emptied normally in less than 4 ½ hours.

It has been found that even a little bit of nibbling delays digestion to the extent that eleven hours after breakfast, there is still a large residue left in the stomach. This sort of routine insults the human mechanism, destroys its normal function, and lessens the efficiency of mind, body, and emotions. Many of the chemicals produced during partial digestion are toxic. These cause an intoxication of brain, liver, kidneys and other delicate tissues. Probably, the key to regularity in eating lies in having a good breakfast. When the morning meal is omitted, one tends to become hungry before noon and resorts to snacking.

The best routine is to eat breakfast within three hours of arising, wait at least five hours (preferably six to seven) before having lunch. Again, wait five hours before supper, and have a light supper of fruit and grains, taken several hours before bedtime. (Thrash 2013)

It is best to omit the third meal. It is our hope that it will become your habit during this program. It will give you extra strength and save on the food bill, too!

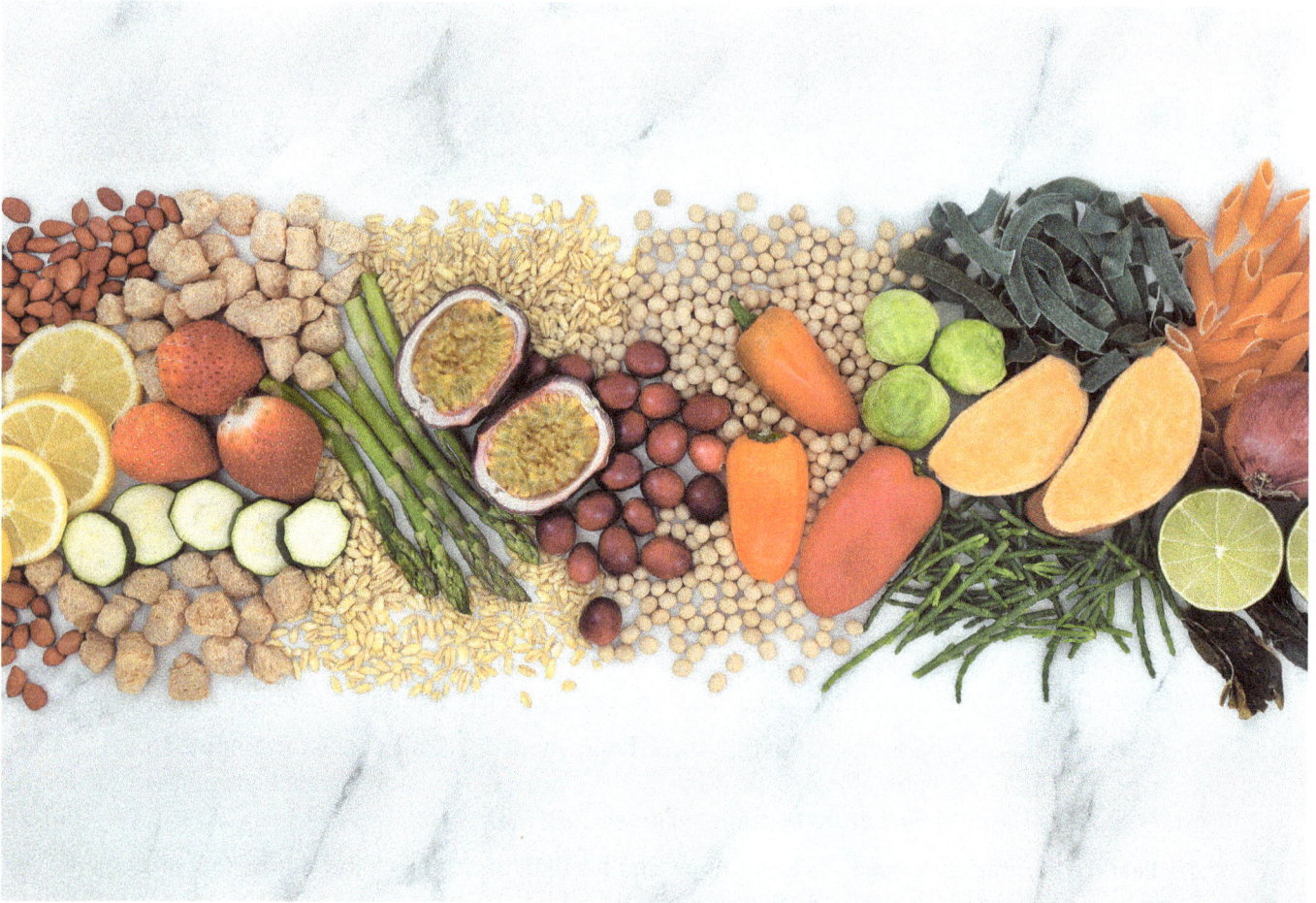

Physical Awareness

MORE ABOUT HEALTHY FOODS AND GOD'S FOOD RESTORATION

POLYSACCHARIDES: Polysaccharides are sources of natural sugar found in roots, fruits and grains. Carbohydrates are polysaccharides. Every meal of the day should be planned around a carbohydrate, which includes grains, roots, and starches.

GRAINS: Wheat, rye, spelt, barley, oats, millet, quinoa, buckwheat cereals, brown rice, bulgur wheat, cornmeal, rolled oats, and quick oats, wheat berries, wheat bran, wheat germ

ROOTS: White potatoes, sweet potatoes, pumpkin, beetroots, parsnips, carrots, turnips, cassava, yucca

FLOURS: Buckwheat, gluten, millet, rice, rye, soy, barley, whole wheat, whole wheat pastry

FRUITS: Apples, bananas, grapes, grapefruits, mangoes, pears, melons, oranges, pineapples, plums, strawberries. (The best are Granny Smith apples, grapefruit, lemons, avocado, tomatoes, and limes. Many others can be eaten to your liking.)

GOD'S FOOD RESTORATION

SPICES that have *health restoring* properties are: cayenne pepper, turmeric, ocean salt, basil, oregano, coriander, rosemary, parsley, ginger, and onions.

HEALTHY FATS (oils) include: olives (black in their natural juice), olive oil, coconut oil, flaxseed oil, and coconut cream. Other healthy fats include nuts, avocados, and grains.

The essential fatty acids (EFAs) are:

Omega-3—found in walnuts, chia seeds, flax seeds/oil, soybeans, avocados and turnips.

Omega-6—found in pumpkins, sunflower seeds, corn, olives, flax seeds/oil, tofu or soy, and walnuts.

Note: Make sure the olive oil you buy is extra virgin, cold pressed, and in a dark jar.

HERBS: basil, celery seed, chives, cardamom, coriander, cumin, dill seed, garlic cloves/powder, Italian seasoning, marjoram, onion flakes/powder, orange peel, oregano, paprika, parsley, sage, savory, taco seasoning, thyme, turmeric.

> Using Herbs Medicinally: For bitter herbs, a good rule of thumb is to use them seven days on and seven days off. The more mild herbs can be used every day. Some bitter herbs include, but are not limited to: gentian, yarrow, wormwood, goldenseal, dandelion, chamomile, milk thistle, and echinacea.

FLAVORINGS: Coffee substitute (Cafix®, Pero®, Roma®, etc.), carob powder

EXTRACTS: almond, orange, maple, vanilla, lemon juice, nutritional yeast flakes, natural salt

NATURAL SUGARS/SWEETENERS: You can find natural sugars in fruit, honey, blackstrap molasses, maple syrup, stevia, and sucanat. Stevia is the best sweetener for a diabetic. There is a concern as to whether honey is an animal product, and if vegetarians should eat it (Prov. 24:13; 25:16, 27).

AVOID: High fructose corn syrup, Splenda, aspartame, and white, processed sugar.

SPECIALTY ITEMS: dairy-free milk, soy or tofu powder, vegetable oil, pastas (lasagna, noodles, elbows, veggie spirals), tofu, silken tofu or water pack, active yeast

HEALTHY BACTERIA: should come from sourdough bread, sauerkraut, miso, tofu, tempeh, and yogurt

YOUR CHALLENGES ARE:

__to try to put your own healthy recipe together.

Recipe Name: _____

....

....

....

....

....

....

....

....

....

....

....

....

....

....

__to do a **SECOND MILE ACT** for someone:

__**to claim this promise:** *"He shall call upon me, and I will answer him: I will be with him in trouble; I will deliver him, and honour him. With long life will I satisfy him, and shew him my salvation"* (Ps. 91:15, 16).

RECIPE FOR THE DAY

CHINESE RICE

2½ cups rice (hot)

½ cup celery

⅓ cup sliced mushrooms (optional)

½ cup raw cashews

2 Tbsp. oil

½ tsp. salt

1 small box tofu

SLICE tofu into ½-inch thick pieces and brown lightly on both sides. Add celery, mushrooms and 2 tablespoons water. Simmer until the celery is tender. Add soy sauce and rice. Mix and simmer for 5 minutes.

MENTAL & MORAL AWARENESS

GOD'S ROYAL LAW & COVENANT

Supplemental Reading: *Exodus 20:1–17, Deuteronomy 4:13, James 2:8–12*

#1 of God's Ten Commandments is about loving and serving Him.

"And God spake all these words, saying, I am the LORD thy God, which have brought thee out of the land of Egypt, out of the house of bondage. Thou shalt have no other gods before me" (Ex. 20:1–3).

WHAT DOES THE BIBLE SAY?

How to Keep the Sabbath

- What did Jesus say about the Sabbath *(Ex. 20:8)?*
- How long was each day of Creation *(Gen. 1:23, 31)?*
- When does the Sabbath begin and end *(Lev. 23:32)?*
- What is the preparation day *(Mark 15:42)?*
- Why were the Jews condemned in Nehemiah's time *(Neh. 13:15–22)?*

✓ *DAILY WELLNESS CHECK*

__Am I still forgiving today?

__Am I being thankful today?

__Am I happy today?

__Am I helpful today?

__Am I obedient today?

__Did I eat more fruits and vegetables today?

__Was I intimate with God today?

__Am I ready for bed on time today?

__Did I drink enough water today?

__Did I overdo anything today?

__Did I exercise today?

__Am I taking deep breaths today?

__Did I get enough sunshine today?

__Did I dress appropriately today?

MY PRAYERS & CHALLENGES

....

....

....

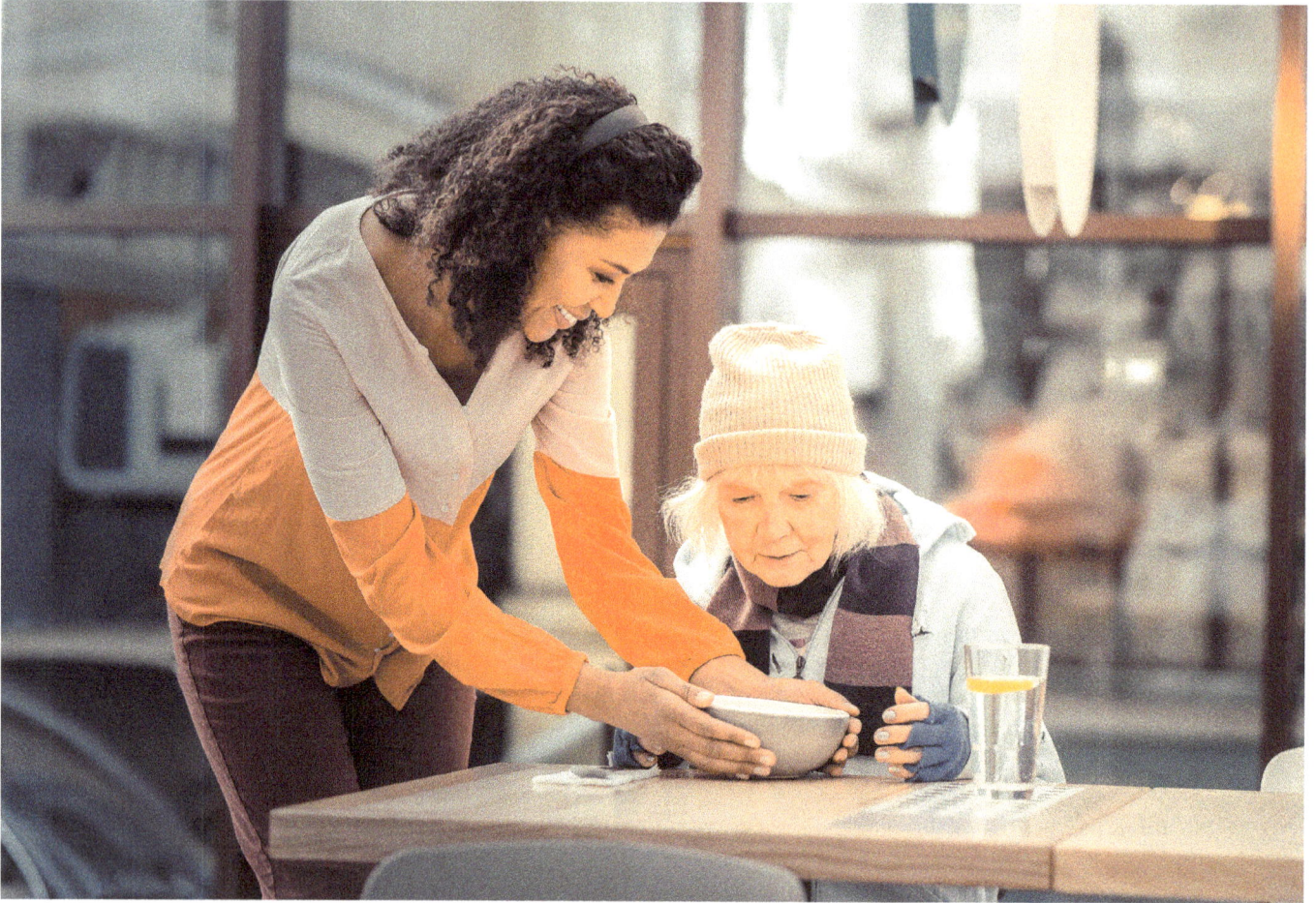

Physical Awareness

A CLOSER LOOK AT INTIMACY WITH GOD

What is He requiring of me?

- A contrite (repentant) heart
- A heart opened to the light of truth
- Love and compassion for my fellow man
- A Spirit refusing to be bribed through avarice or self-love
- To put away every evil habit of disobedience to Him, including my unhealthy eating, drinking, and sleeping habits, etc. (Jer. 31:10–12).

YOUR CHALLENGES ARE:

__to keep worshipping, starting and ending with prayer.

__to keep singing several songs from your hymnal, or ones you wrote yourself.

__to keep randomly opening the Bible and read the first thing you set your heart on; then believe and receive it as a promise or as an answer to a problem you are having.

__to keep praying sincerely. Keep using the text that you studied in your prayer. Stay genuine when you are praying and while remaining humble and reverent.

__to keep remembering that you are talking (praying) to your Father and Savior who also wants to be your friend.

__to do a **SECOND MILE ACT** for someone:

__**to claim this promise:** *"For I the Lord thy God will hold thy right hand, saying unto thee, Fear not; I will help thee"* (Isa. 41:13).

RECIPE FOR THE DAY

STIR FRY VEGETABLES

6 small, fresh squash (sliced)

6 small, fresh zucchini (sliced)

1 lb. fresh okra (sliced)

3 whole corn on the cob (sliced cork wheel)

1 red bell pepper (sliced)

1 green bell pepper (sliced)

½ bunch of green onions

Oil and seasoning to taste

HEAT a skillet with a tablespoon of soybean oil. Add the above vegetables to skillet and stir for 15–20 minutes, or until brown.

MENTAL & MORAL AWARENESS

GOD'S ROYAL LAW & COVENANT

Supplemental Reading: Exodus 20:1–17, Deuteronomy 4:13, James 2:8–12

#2 of God's 10 Commandments is about loving and serving Him.

Thou shalt not make unto thee any graven image, or any likeness of anything that is in heaven above, or that is in the earth beneath, or that is in the water under the earth: thou shalt not bow down thyself to them, nor serve them: for I the LORD thy God am a jealous God, visiting the iniquity of the fathers upon the children unto the third and fourth generation of them that hate me: And shewing mercy unto thousands of them that love me, and keep my commandments (see Matt. 4:10; Acts 24:14).

WHAT DOES THE BIBLE SAY?

How to Keep the Sabbath

- What should we do on the Sabbath *(Isa. 58:13, 14)?*

- What day did Jesus worship on *(Luke 4:16)?*
- Should we help others on the Sabbath *(Matt. 12:10–13)?*
- What is God's special sign to His people *(Ezek. 20:12, 20)?*

✓ *DAILY WELLNESS CHECK*

__*Am I still forgiving today?*

__*Am I being thankful today?*

__*Am I happy today?*

__*Am I helpful today?*

__*Am I obedient today?*

__*Did I eat more fruits and vegetables today?*

__*Was I intimate with God today?*

__*Am I ready for bed on time today?*

__*Did I drink enough water today?*

__*Did I overdo anything today?*

__*Did I exercise today?*

__*Am I taking deep breaths today?*

__*Did I get enough sunshine today?*

__*Did I dress appropriately today?*

MY PRAYERS & CHALLENGES

....

....

....

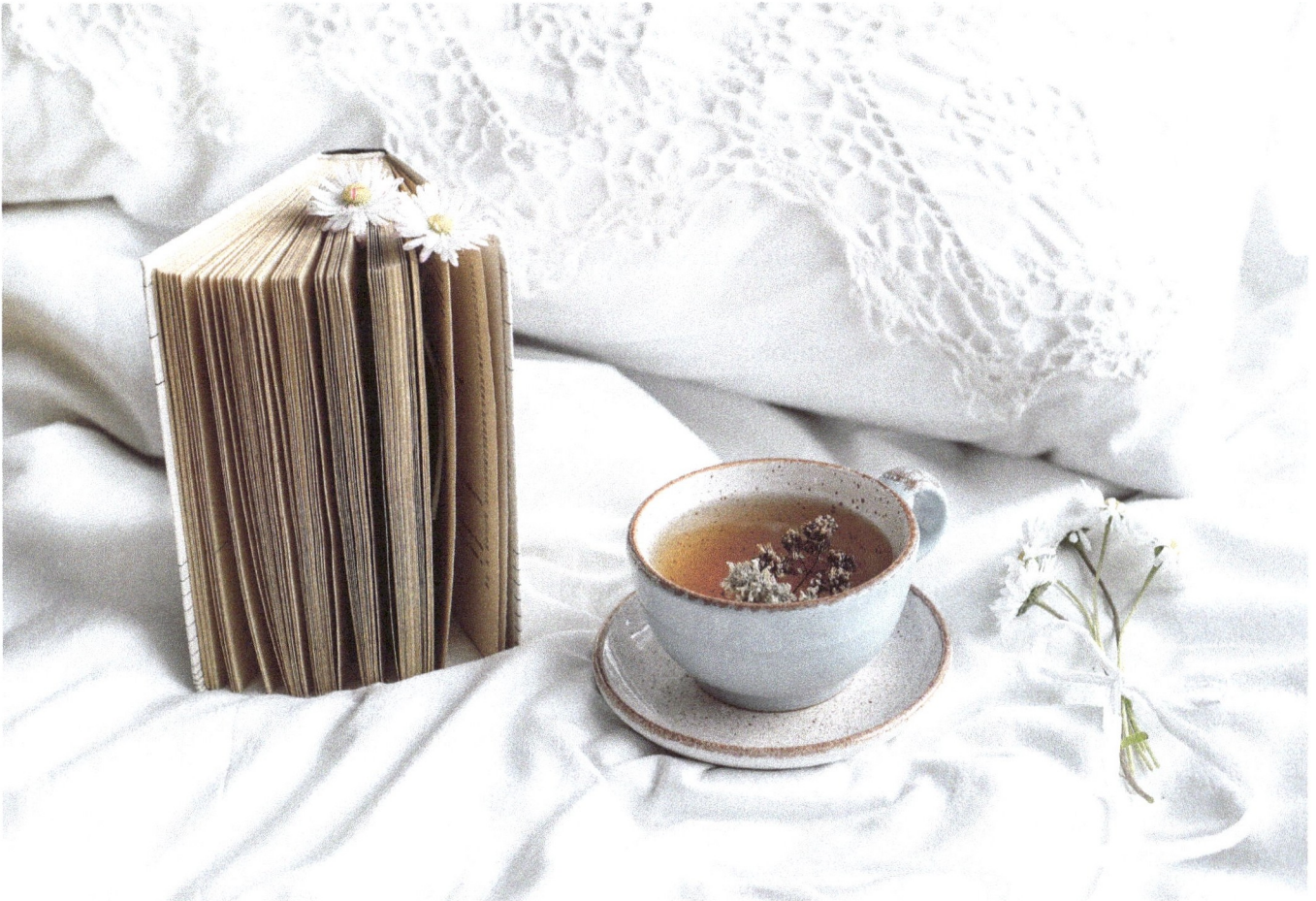

Physical Awareness

MORE FACTS ABOUT SLEEP

- When the body is deprived of sleep, it is unable to rebuild and recharge itself adequately.
- Without sufficient sleep, there is an increase in irritability, while creativity, concentration, and efficiency suffer.
- Sleep deprivation impairs judgement, causing values and priorities to change.
- Continued loss of sleep can result in exhaustion, depression, delusions, paranoia, and hallucinations.
- Losing even a single night of sleep can cut the effectiveness of your immune system in half.
- Slowed reaction time and decreased concentration leads to an increased risk of accidents, both fatal and nonfatal.
- Estimates suggest that twenty-one percent of fatal automobile accidents are caused by a driver falling asleep at the wheel ("Facts Statistics: Drowsy Driving").

- In a classic health study, it was found that people who regularly slept seven to eight hours each night had lower death rates than those who slept fewer hours than that.

- "Those who sleep 9 HOURS have a HIGHER MORTALITY rate than those who sleep 7 or 8 hours. During sleep the body is continually at work. It REBUILDS its TISSUES and ALKALINIZES ITSELF; BURNS UP STORED ENERGY; PRODUCES POISONOUS WASTES; and REPAIRS CELLS and TISSUES. BRAIN WORKERS require more sleep than others" (Paulien 1997, p. 109).

- Everyone should put their feet up for half an hour every day after work, or after the day's activity.

YOUR CHALLENGES ARE:

__to increase your exercise program. It will calm the nerves, relax the muscles, and rest the mind.

__to drink relaxing herbal teas. Chamomile, valerian, hops, or passionflower are great choices.

__to avoid caffeine and nicotine.

__to do a **SECOND MILE ACT** for someone:

__**to claim this promise:** *"yet will I not forget thee"* (Isa. 49:15).

RECIPE FOR THE DAY

LENTIL-TOMATO LOAF

1 lb. lentils (cooked, drained lentils take 30–35 min. to cook)

2 cups tomato puree or soup

½ cup onions, sautéed

½ cup celery, sautéed

2 tsp. salt

1 clove garlic, minced

½ tsp. thyme

4 slices bread, crumbled

2 Tbsp. oil

MIX bread with tomato soup or puree. Add lentils cooked to almost dry with onions, celery, and the rest of the ingredients. Mix well and bake in loaf pan at 350 degrees for 45 minutes or until set. This makes great leftover sandwiches.

MENTAL & MORAL AWARENESS

GOD'S ROYAL LAW & COVENANT

Supplemental reading: Exodus 20:1–17, Deuteronomy 4:13, James 2:8–12

#3 of God's 10 Commandments is about loving and serving Him

"Thou shalt not take the name of the LORD thy God in vain: for the LORD will not hold him guiltless that taketh his name in vain" (Ex. 20:7).

WHAT DOES THE BIBLE SAY?

Judgment

- Will all people be judged by God (*Acts 17:30, 31*)?

- What about those who love God (*Eccles. 3:17*)?
- Does God have a record of our lives (*Eccles. 12:14*)?
- How does God record our lives (*Dan. 7:9, 10*)?

✓ *DAILY WELLNESS CHECK*

__Am I still forgiving today?

__Am I being thankful today?

__Am I happy today?

__Am I helpful today?

__Am I obedient today?

__Did I eat more fruits and vegetables today?

__Was I intimate with God today?

__Am I ready for bed on time today?

__Did I drink enough water today?

__Did I overdo anything today?

__Did I exercise today?

__Am I taking deep breaths today?

__Did I get enough sunshine today?

__Did I dress appropriately today

MY PRAYERS & CHALLENGES

……

……

……

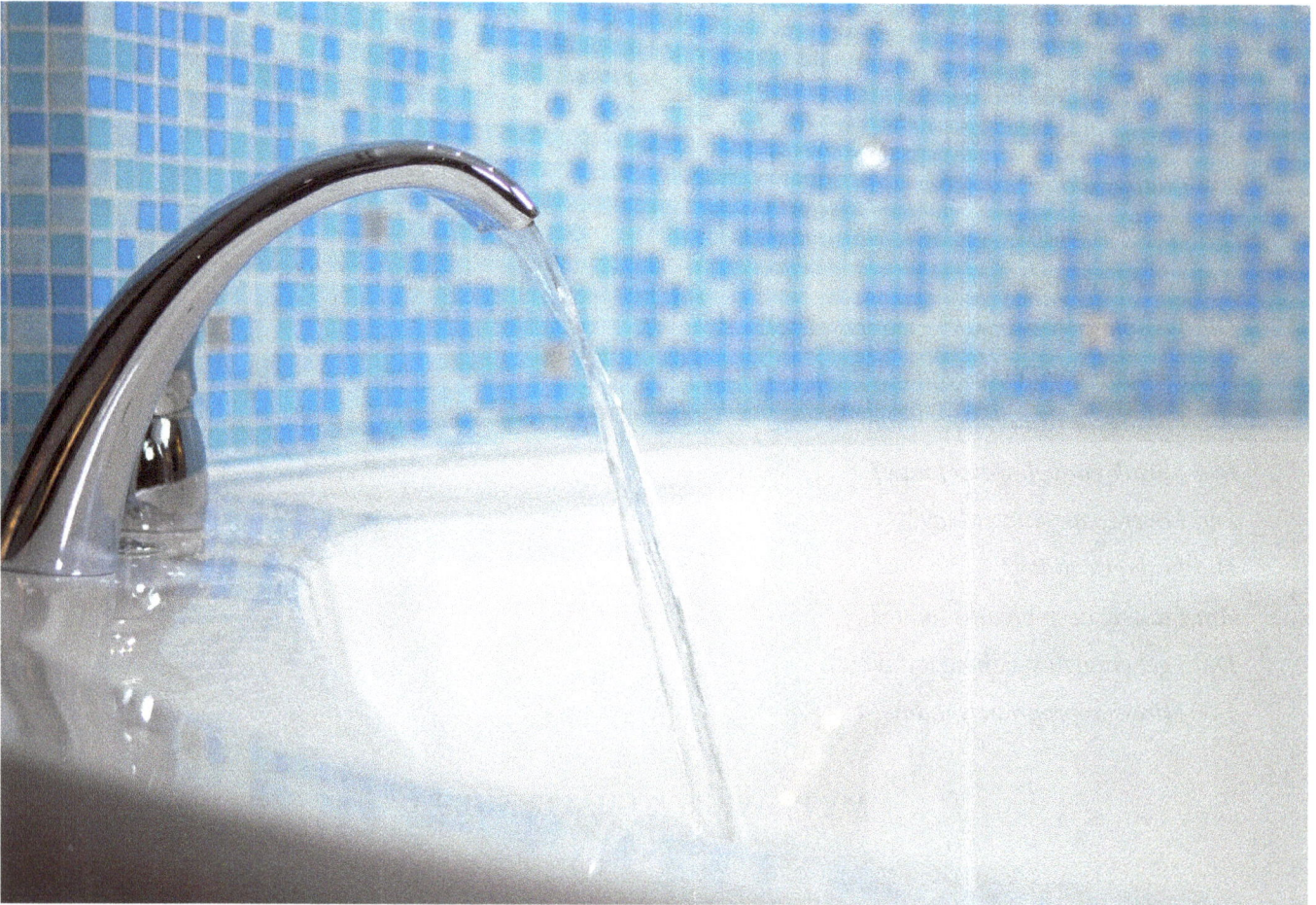

Physical Awareness

MORE FACTS ABOUT WATER

- The skin needs to be cleansed daily from waste material that is given off through the pores. If this is not done, the body will reabsorb these toxic waste materials.

- Water is needed to lubricate and cushion the bones and joints, and to moisten the eyes.

- Water is necessary for the production of saliva and digestive juices.

- Taking a shower or bath will rid the body of odors.

- A bath or shower will improve circulation and invigorate the body.

- To avoid constipation problems, drink your required amount of water daily. The fiber and water together will jointly assist in eliminating waste products that build up in the system.

YOUR CHALLENGES ARE:

__to drink three to four quarts of water a day.

To help you **lose at least a pound per day:**

Drink the first and the last quart in twenty minutes, and at room temperature. Sip on the two remaining quarts during the middle of the day in order to avoid dehydration. Let the first quart in the morning be warm or hot, and add lemon juice. The lemon will help expel gas, boost liver function, clean the stomach, break up excess uric acid in joints that causes pain, and help you have a good bowel movement.

__to do a **SECOND MILE ACT** for someone:

__**to claim this promise:** *"There hath not failed one word of all his good promise"* (1 Kings 8:56).

RECIPE FOR THE DAY

WHEAT GARDEN TABOULI SALAD

1 cup bulgur wheat

1 cup boiling water

¼ cup olive oil

⅓ cup lemon juice

1 tsp. salt

¼ tsp. garlic powder

¼ cup onions chopped

½ tsp. oregano leaves (optional)

1 large tomato, chopped

2 ½ oz. black olives, canned, sliced

In medium bowl, POUR boiling water over bulgur wheat. Let sit for half an hour. Mix in shaker oil, lemon juice, salt, garlic powder, oregano; shake well. Mix bulgur wheat and vegetables; pour in seasoning mixture and stir well. Serve over bed of lettuce or in pita pocket.

MENTAL & MORAL AWARENESS

GOD'S ROYAL LAW & COVENANT

Supplemental Reading: Exodus 20:1–17, Deuteronomy 4:13, James 2:8–12

#4 of God's 10 Commandments is about loving and serving Him.

"Remember the Sabbath day, to keep it holy. Six days shalt thou labor, and do all thy work: But the seventh day is the sabbath of the LORD thy God: in it thou shalt not do any work, thou, nor thy son, nor thy daughter, thy manservant, nor thy maidservant, nor thy cattle, nor thy stranger that is within thy gates: For in six days the LORD made heaven and earth, the sea, and all that in them is, and rested the seventh day: wherefore the LORD blessed the sabbath day, and hallowed it" (Ex. 20:8–11).

WHAT DOES THE BIBLE SAY?

Judgment

• Whose names will not be blotted out of the book of life *(Rev. 3:5)?*

- How are we judged *(Rev. 20:12)?*
- What is God's reward *(Rev. 22:12)?*
- What is the difference between the sheep and the goats *(Matt. 25:25–41)?*

✓ *DAILY WELLNESS CHECK*

__*Am I still forgiving today?*

__*Am I being thankful today?*

__*Am I happy today?*

__*Am I helpful today?*

__*Am I obedient today?*

__*Did I eat more fruits and vegetables today?*

__*Was I intimate with God today?*

__*Am I ready for bed on time today?*

__*Did I drink enough water today?*

__*Did I overdo anything today?*

__*Did I exercise today?*

__*Am I taking deep breaths today?*

__*Did I get enough sunshine today?*

__*Did I dress appropriately today*

MY PRAYERS & CHALLENGES

....

....

....

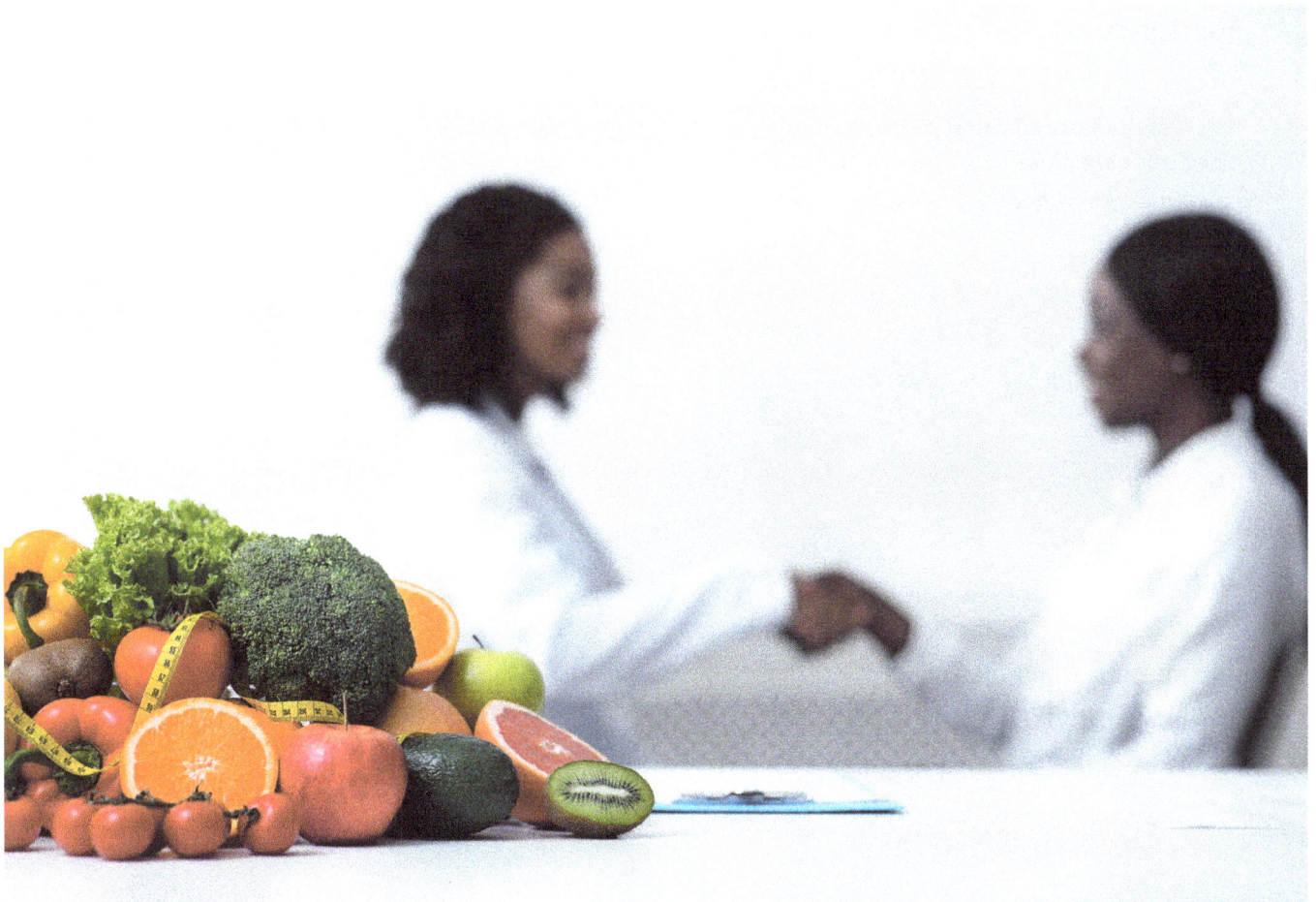

Physical Awareness

MORE ABOUT TEMPERANCE ALWAYS

MILK—of another species is not natural for humans to consume. Drinking milk after being weaned from our mother's milk is not natural either. Milk consumption increases allergies such as hay fever. Cheese increases allergies, causes constipation, and affects neuro-transmitter levels in the brain.

SUGAR—robs the body of B vitamins. It has no nutrients but requires nutrients to digest. It suppresses the immune system. The average American eats over 100 pounds of sugar per year! Sugar contains no fiber. Fiber regulates the rate at which sugar enters the blood stream.

SODAS—contain high concentrations of white sugar. They also often contain high fructose corn syrup, which increase appetite. The average child drinks 800 cans of soda per year. Soda ends up being 20% of a child's caloric intake! Sodas will cause a decrease in intellect and energy. They will excite the nervous system, which results in depression.

CHOCOLATE—contains caffeine, which is addictive and is associated with higher levels of breast and colon cancer. It contains theobromine, which is a stimulant. Astonishingly, it may have rodent dung or hairs, and insect fragments. The USDA allows at least 10 milligrams per pound of visible or solid animal excretion, and up to 120 insect fragments per cup.

YOUR CHALLENGES ARE:

__to eat only two meals per day. (This will help with weight loss because your body will feed off itself at night.)

__to do a **SECOND MILE ACT** for someone:

__**to claim this promise:** *"Is any sick among you? Let him call for the elders of the church; and let them pray over him, anointing him with oil in the name of the Lord: And the prayer of faith shall save the sick, and the Lord shall raise him up; and if he have committed sins, they shall be forgiven him"* (James 5:14, 15).

RECIPE FOR THE DAY

POTATO CHEESE

2 cups boiled potatoes

1½ cups water

2 Tbsp. garlic powder

1 tsp. salt

⅓ cup oil

⅓ cup celery

½ cup nutritional yeast flakes

¼ cup pimentos (or cooked carrots)

BLEND together. Serve hot or cold.

MENTAL & MORAL AWARENESS

MORE FACTS ABOUT FORGIVENESS

- Forgiveness must be sincerely from the heart. The pretense of forgiveness motivated by circumstances or by ulterior motives may deceive the one being forgiven, but it will never deceive God, who looks on the heart.

- Humans naturally rely on feelings, but God deals with principle, so rehearse the principle of forgiveness in the Bible: (1) 1 John 1:9 , "If we confess our sins, he is faithful and just to forgive us our sins, and to cleanse us from all unrighteousness;" (2) Mark 11:26, "But if ye do not forgive , neither will your Father which is in heaven forgive your trespasses" . Meditate on these promises and see God change your attitude.

WHAT DOES THE BIBLE SAY?

Healthful Living

- Is God concerned about eating and drinking *(1 Cor. 10:31)*?

- What is your body *(1 Cor. 6:19, 20)*?

- What was man's original diet *(Gen. 1:29, 30)*?

- When did vegetables begin to grow *(Gen. 3:18)*?

✓ *DAILY WELLNESS CHECK*

__Am I still forgiving today?

__Am I being thankful today?

__Am I happy today?

__Am I helpful today?

__Am I obedient today?

__Did I eat more fruits and vegetables today?

__Was I intimate with God today?

__Am I ready for bed on time today?

__Did I drink enough water today?

__Did I overdo anything today?

__Did I exercise today?

__Am I taking deep breaths today?

__Did I get enough sunshine today?

__Did I dress appropriately today?

MY PRAYERS & CHALLENGES

....

....

....

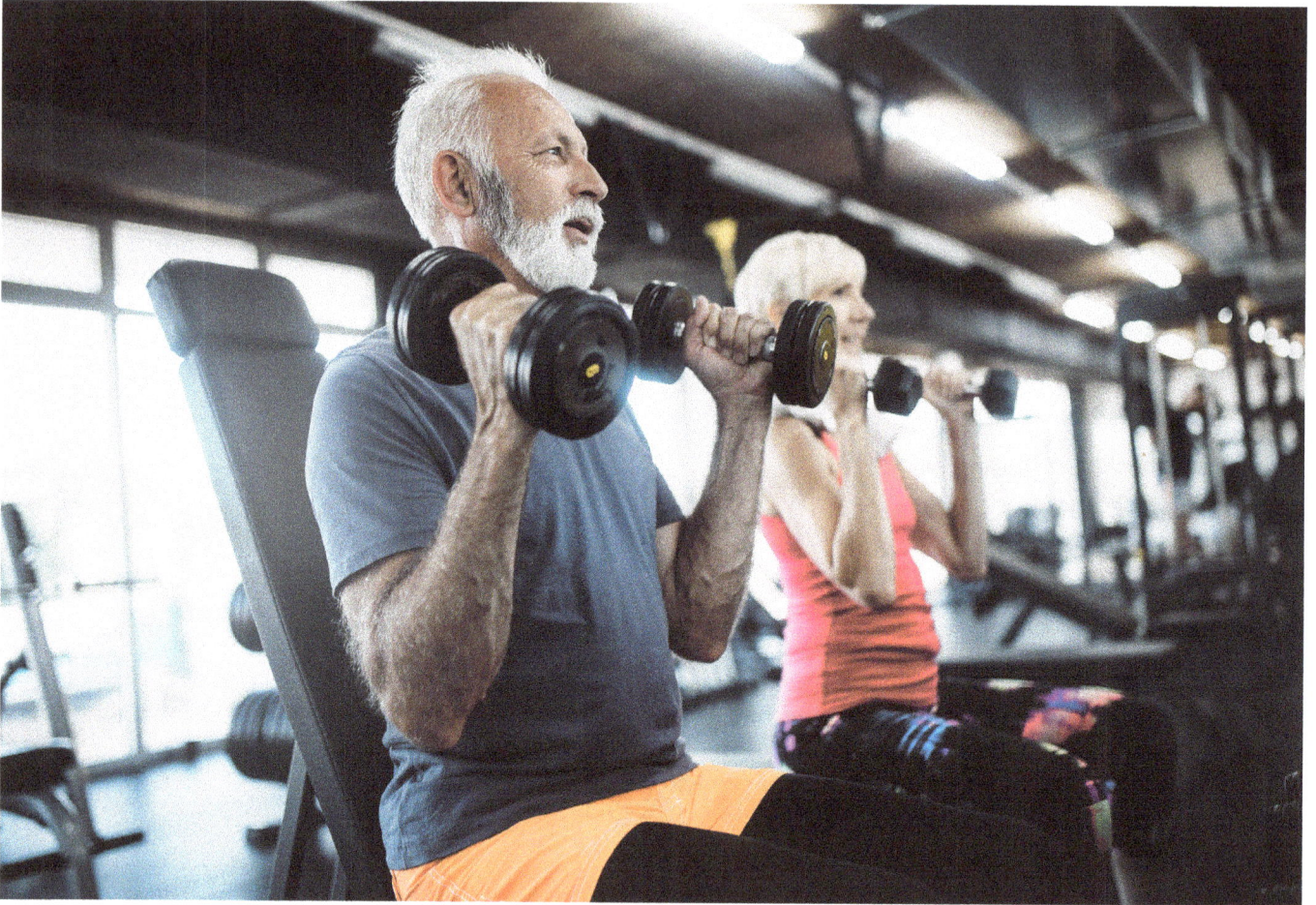

Physical Awareness

MORE FACTS ABOUT DAILY EXERCISE

- Muscle tone is developed by exercise. Good resistance exercises like weight training and sit-ups, are perfect to burn fat and reshape the body.

- Exercise reduces stress, tension, and depression, and creates a happy state of mind by increasing the production of norepinephrine activity in the brain.

- It will make your mind more alert.

- It increases longevity.

- It aids digestion.

- It helps promote sleep.

- It increases bone density.

- It strengthens the immune system.

YOUR CHALLENGES ARE:

__to increase your exercise program. (For good health maintenance, walk for thirty minutes a day; for health restoration, walk for sixty minutes a day. This routine is proven to assist your body with building definition, building muscles, losing weight, and improving your outlook on life.)

__to do a **SECOND MILE ACT** for someone:

__**to claim this promise:** *"If thou will diligently hearken to the voice of the LORD they God, and wilt do that which is right in his sight, and wilt give ear to his commandments, and keep all his statures, I will put none of these diseases upon thee, which I have brought upon the Egyptians: for I am the LORD that healeth thee"* (Ex. 15:26).

RECIPE FOR THE DAY

LESSARRELLA CHEESE

2 cups water

¼ cup cornstarch

⅓ cup quick oats

¼ cup tahini

1/4 cup sunflower seeds (optional for thicker cheese)

½ cup yeast flakes

3 Tbsp. lemon juice

1 Tbsp. onion powder

1½ tsp. salt

BLEND until smooth. Pour into saucepan and cook on medium, stirring constantly until thickened. Heat for macaroni and cheese, or pour into any molding pan and chill overnight. Can be sliced. Delicious on crackers, pizza or in sandwiches. May sprinkle on herbs and melt under broiler.

MENTAL & MORAL AWARENESS

MORE FACTS ABOUT THANKFULNESS

- Forget your own difficulties and troubles, and praise God for an opportunity to live for the glory of His name.
- Let the fresh blessings of each new day awaken praise in our hearts for these tokens of His loving care. When you open your eyes in the morning, thank God that He has kept you through the night. Thank Him for His peace in your heart. **Morning, noon, and night**, let gratitude ascend to heaven as a sweet perfume.
- Do not talk of your lack of faith or your sorrows and sufferings. The tempter, the enemy of our souls, delights to hear such words. When you talk about gloomy subjects, you glorify the enemy. We are not to dwell on the power of Satan to overcome us. We often give ourselves into his hands by talking of his power.
- Let us talk instead of the **great power of God** to bind up all our interests with His own. Talk of the matchless power of Christ and His glory.

THE CHALLENGE IS:

__to meditate on what you study. Meditate also on the closing scenes of Jesus' life by reading Matthew 27:11–54, or Isaiah 53 and keep a THANKFUL spirit.

WHAT DOES THE BIBLE SAY?

Healthful Living

- When did man begin to eat flesh *(Gen. 9:3, 4)?*
- Is all flesh clean *(Deut. 14:1–20)?*
- Is strong drink good for a Christian *(Prov. 20:1)?*
- What is God's plan for our lives *(3 John 2)?*

✓ *DAILY WELLNESS CHECK*

__Am I still forgiving today?

__Am I being thankful today?

__Am I happy today?

__Am I helpful today?

__Am I obedient today?

__Did I eat more fruits and vegetables today?

__Was I intimate with God today?

__Am I ready for bed on time today?

__Did I drink enough water today?

__Did I overdo anything today?

__Did I exercise today?

__Am I taking deep breaths today?

__Did I get enough sunshine today?

__Did I dress appropriately today?

MY PRAYERS & CHALLENGES

....

....

....

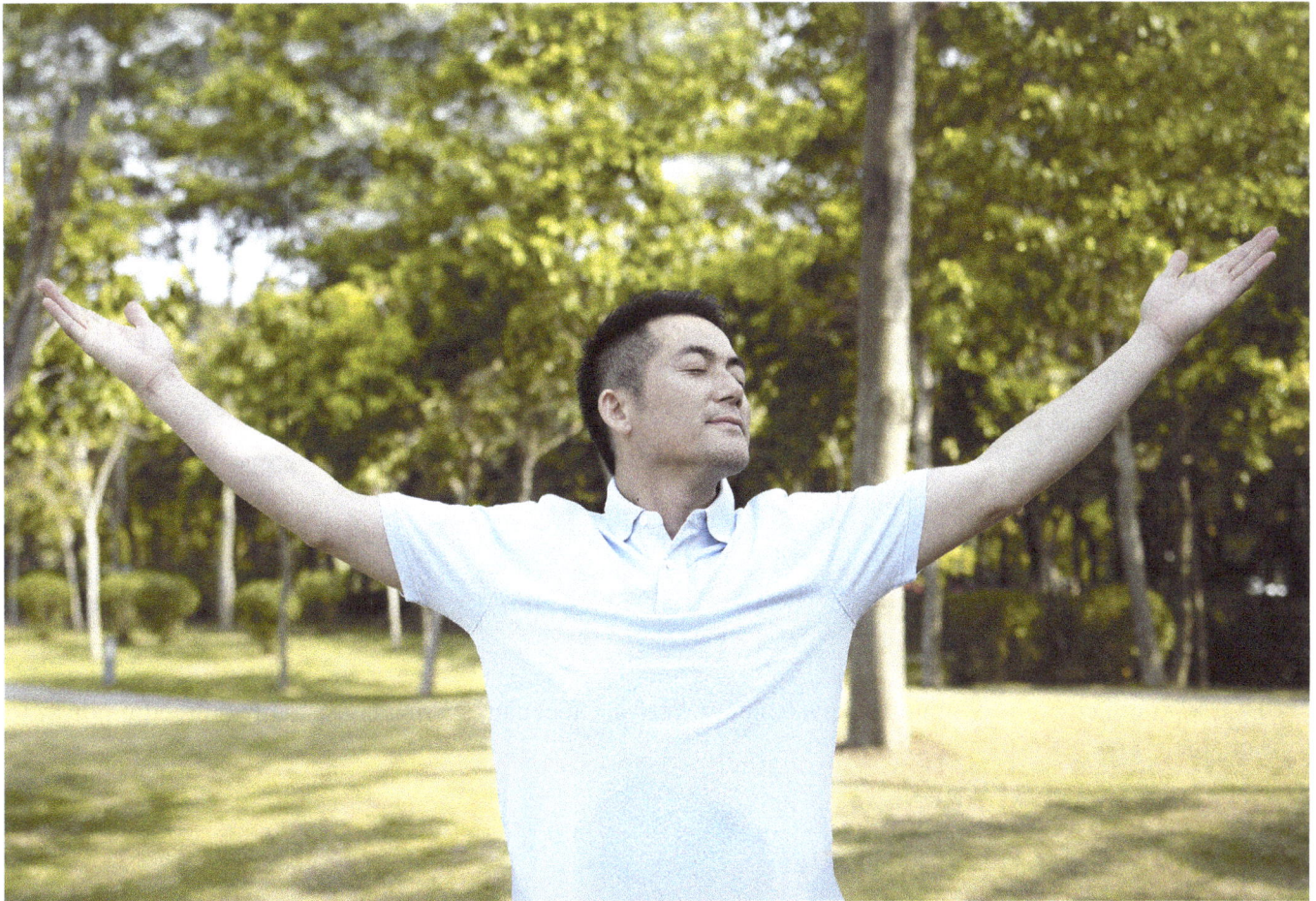

Physical Awareness

MORE FACTS ABOUT PURE, FRESH AIR

How to Breathe

The following breathing exercises will help expel impure air from the lungs and let in pure, fresh air. For better breathing, concentrate less on inhalation and more on exhalation. The more air you breathe out or exhale, the more air you can breathe in or inhale.

1. Breathe in through the nose to the count of 4.
2. After a pause on the count of 7, breathe out slowly to the count of 9.
3. Increase the time by breathing in to the count of 5, pause to the count of 7, then breathing out to the count of 15.
4. Gradually increase the depth of each exhalation until you can exhale to the count of 30 or more.
5. Practice deep breathing exercises (10–20 deep breaths) several times a day.

Do this if you are feeling ill, fatigued, anxious, stressed, or have a headache.

YOUR CHALLENGES ARE:

__to avoid staying in the house all day.

__to do a **SECOND MILE ACT** for someone:

__**to claim this promise:** *"Lord…heal my soul; for I have sinned against thee"* (Ps. 41:4).

RECIPE FOR THE DAY

AMERICAN or NUT CHEESE

1 cup water

1 cup cashews OR any nut

2 Tbsp. sesame seeds

3 Tbsp. nutritional yeast flakes

1 tsp. onion powder

¼ tsp. garlic powder

1 tsp. salt

½ cup steamed carrot

2 Tbsp. lemon juice

BLEND until completely smooth. Serve cold, or heat in saucepan, stirring consistently on medium heat to thicken; then serve.

MENTAL & MORAL AWARENESS

MORE FACTS ON HOW TO LOVE LIFE

- Spending time outdoors in the sunshine and fresh air nourishes the brain and fills the eyes with wondrous sites of nature that provide a sense of peaceful contentment.
- Do not look to yourself or others for your joy. Joy comes only from God, Who loves you more than you love yourself, and more than others love you. He loves you even more than a parent or a spouse can love you.
- Fix your eyes on Jesus Christ your Lord and Savior. Remember that weeping may endure for a night, but joy comes in the morning (Ps. 30:5).

THE CHALLENGE IS:

__to write a one-page love letter to your Father in heaven. Pour out your heart to Him.

WHAT DOES THE BIBLE SAY?

Mark of the Beast

- What is the seal of God *(Ex. 20:8–11)?*
- Why do we keep the Sabbath *(Ex. 31:17, 13)?*
- Where can the seal be found *(Rev. 7:2, 3)?*

- Who will be sealed *(Rev 14:1, 5)?*
- What does the third angel's message say *(Rev. 14:9–13)?*

✓ *DAILY WELLNESS CHECK*

__Am I still forgiving today?*

__Am I being thankful today?*

__Am I happy today?*

__Am I helpful today?*

__Am I obedient today?*

__Did I eat more fruits and vegetables today?*

__Was I intimate with God today?*

__Am I ready for bed on time today?*

__Did I drink enough water today?*

__Did I overdo anything today?*

__Did I exercise today?*

__Am I taking deep breaths today?*

__Did I get enough sunshine today?*

__Did I dress appropriately today?*

MY PRAYERS & CHALLENGES

....

....

....

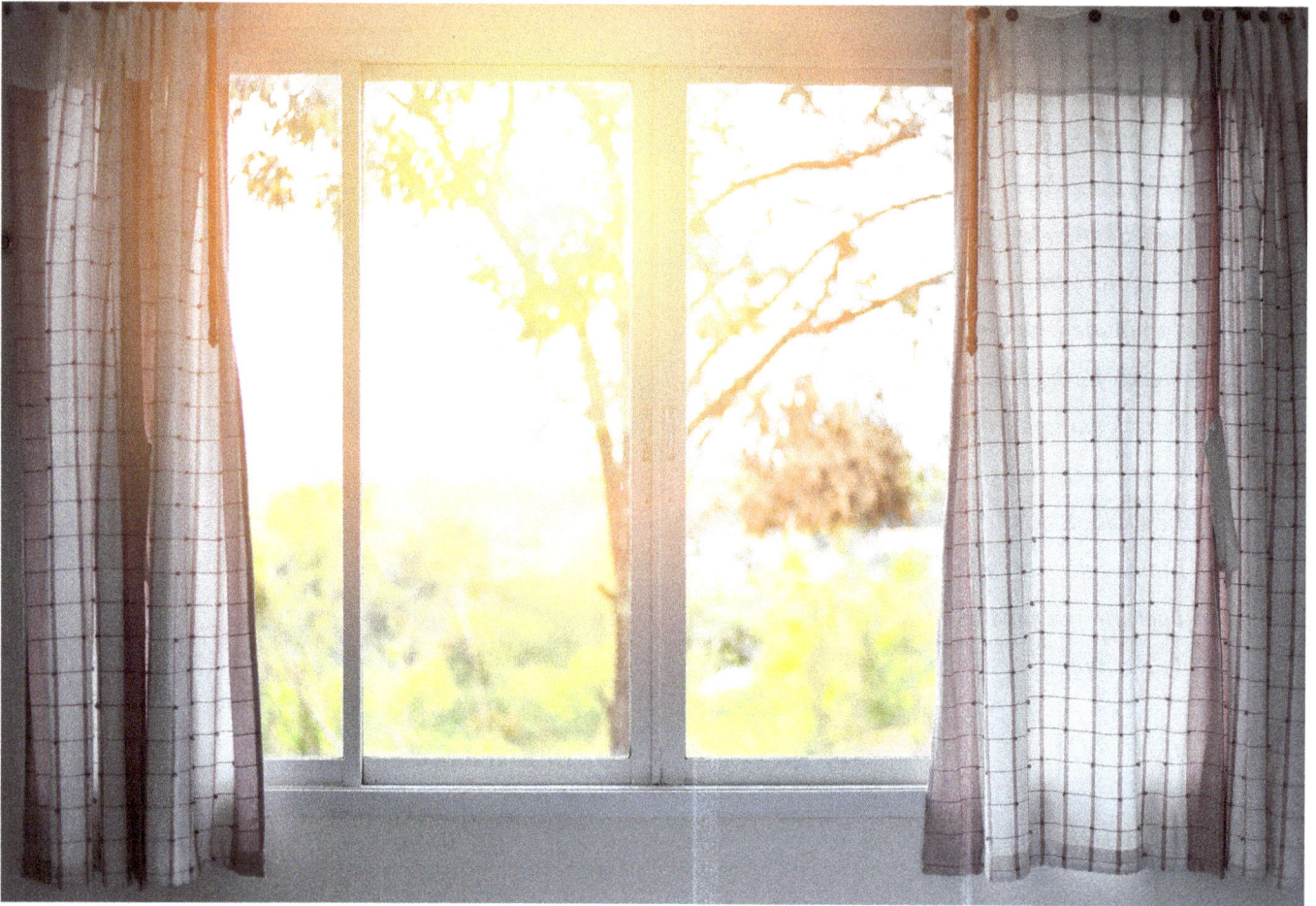

Physical Awareness

MORE FACTS ABOUT SUNLIGHT

- Combined with exercise, it is one of the greatest sleep-inducer.
- It stimulates your appetite and improves your digestion, elimination, and metabolism.
- It improves your complexion.
- To avoid burning the skin and the risk of skin cancer reduce the free fat intake, such as oils, margarine, and other similar foods.
- Our homes need the sunlight to kill germs, especially in our bedrooms.

YOUR CHALLENGES ARE:

__to start doing some outside work or sit on the porch for thirty minutes a day.

__to do a **SECOND MILE ACT** for someone:

__to claim this promise: *"And said, If thou wilt diligently hearken to the voice of the LORD thy God, and wilt do that which is right in his sight, and wilt give ear to his commandments, and keep all his statues, I will put none of these diseases upon thee, which I have brought upon the Egyptians: for I am the LORD that healeth thee"* (Ex. 15:26).

RECIPES FOR THE DAY

SALAD DRESSING

½ cup sunflower seeds

1 cup rice/nut milk

1 tsp. sea salt

½ celery stalk

1 small onion

2 cloves garlic

3 sprigs fresh basil/parsley

3 Tbsp. fresh lemon juice

2 Tbsp. honey or to taste

BLEND until smooth and creamy.

SALAD DRESSINGS MIXES

Can add:

* sesame seeds with paprika and onion powder.

* or sunflower seeds with rice/nut milk, celery, onion, and garlic.

* or tomato paste, relish, basil/parsley, and honey.

* or mayonnaise (veggie mayo) with nutritional yeast and salt.

* or avocado plus basic salad dressing; salt to taste and blend all ingredients until creamy.

MENTAL & MORAL AWARENESS

MORE FACTS ON HOW TO LEND A HELPING HAND

According to Isaiah 58:6-9, the Lord says:

Give your bread to the hungry,

Bring the poor into your house,

Cover the naked,

Help your own flesh or family

Then you shall light up in the morning,

*And your **health** will recover speedily:*

And your righteousness shall be seen;

And the glory of the Lord shall be

your reward.

Then you shall call on God

And He will answer.

WHAT DOES THE BIBLE SAY?

Mark of the Beast

- What is the image to the beast *(Rev. 13:15–18)?*
- What are the two great powers *(Rev. 12:17)?*
- Who will win the battle *(Rev. 15:2)?*
- What is the final fate of the beast *(Rev. 20:10)?*

✓ *DAILY WELLNESS CHECK*

__Am I still forgiving today?__

__Am I being thankful today?__

__Am I happy today?__

__Am I helpful today?__

__Am I obedient today?__

__Did I eat more fruits and vegetables today?__

__Was I intimate with God today?__

__Am I ready for bed on time today?__

__Did I drink enough water today?__

__Did I overdo anything today?__

__Did I exercise today?__

__Am I taking deep breaths today?__

__Did I get enough sunshine today?__

__Did I dress appropriately today?__

MY PRAYERS & CHALLENGES

....

....

....

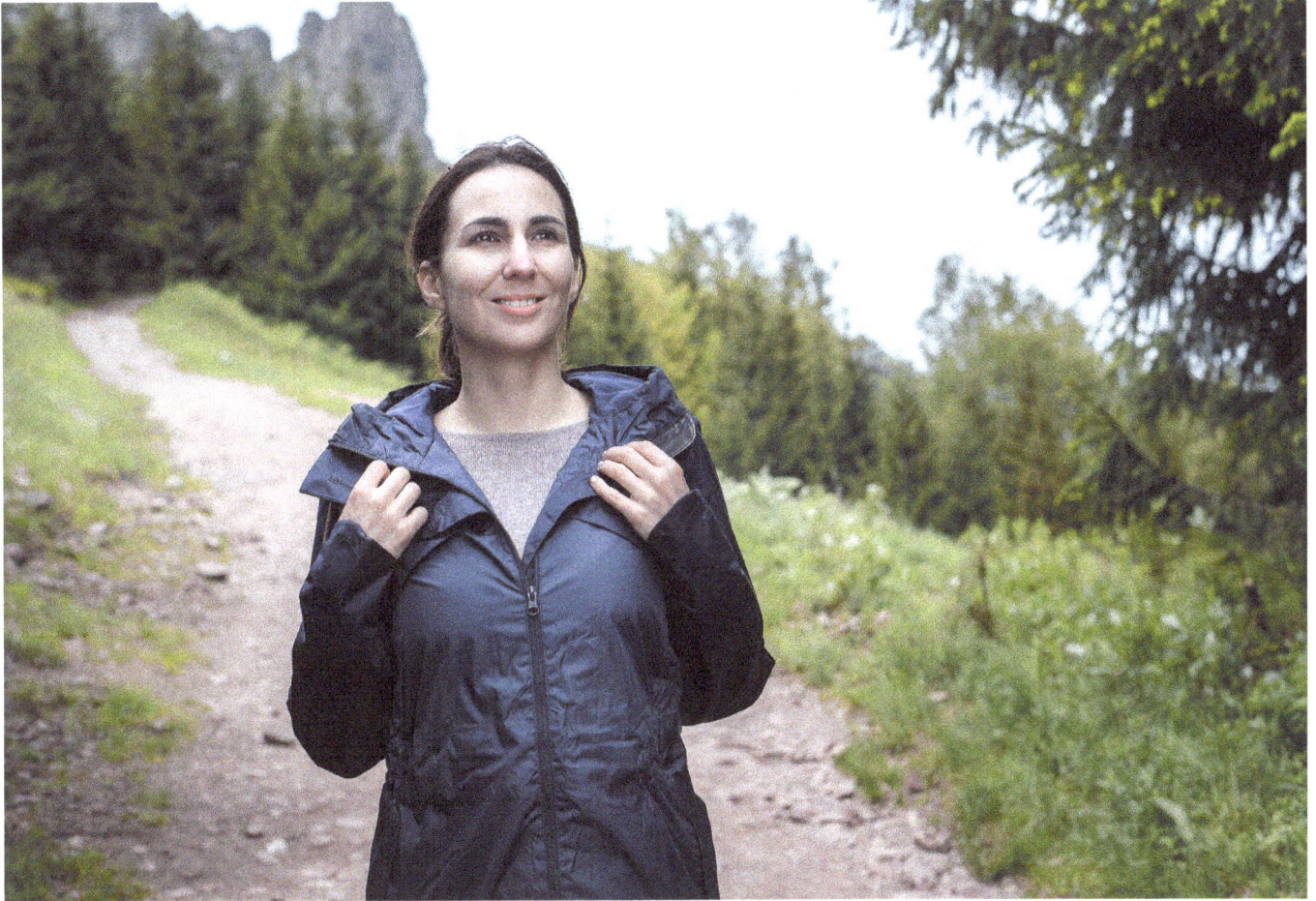

Physical Awareness

MORE FACTS ABOUT WEARING CLOTHES TO PROMOTE HEALTH

- Dress should have the grace, beauty, and appropriateness of natural simplicity. Christ has warned us against the pride of life, but not against its grace and natural beauty. He pointed to the flowers of the field, to the lily unfolding in its purity, and said, *"Even Solomon in all his glory was not arrayed like one of these" (Matt. 6:29).* Thus by the things of nature, Christ illustrates the beauty that heaven values, the modest grace, the simplicity, the purity, the appropriateness, that would make our attire pleasing to Him.

- The most beautiful dress that He bids us to wear is upon the soul. No outward adorning can compare in value or loveliness with that of a "meek and quiet spirit" which in His sight is "of great price" (1 Peter 3:4).

- It was the adversary of all good who instigated the invention of the ever-changing fashions. He desires nothing so much as to bring grief and dishonor to God by working for the misery and ruin of human beings. One of the means by which the enemy most effectually accomplishes the ruin of human beings is through the devices of fashion, which weakens the body, enfeebles the mind, and belittles the soul.

YOUR CHALLENGES ARE:

__to simplify your wardrobe.

__to give something away from your wardrobe.

__to do a **SECOND MILE ACT** for someone:

__**to claim this promise:** *"Bless the Lord, O my soul: and forget not all His benefits: Who forgiveth all thine iniquities; who healeth all thy diseases"* (Ps. 103:2, 3).

RECIPES FOR THE DAY

MASTER CLEANSE

1 quart of water

3 lemons (½ cup juice)

¼ cup maple syrup

⅛ tsp. cayenne pepper

Drink between meals when hungry. (**If you fast and drink this, you can lose 2–3 pounds a day.**)

TIPS FOR MENU PLANNING

• Plan your menu for a week.

• Develop a shopping list.

• Shop by your list.

• Shop after you have had breakfast or lunch.

• Select the best quality of fresh things; stock up only for a week.

• Plan to use leftovers within one to two days. Overall, the diet should consist of 80% complex carbohydrates, 10% fat, and 10% protein.

MENTAL & MORAL AWARENESS

FACTS ABOUT OBEYING WILLINGLY

• God can increase your faith and give you a willing heart if you ask Him (Matt. 7:7).

• Stepping out in faith and being willing to try whatever He asks you to do pleases Him and gives you favor with Him.

• Obeying all of God's Ten Commandments, as He asks, makes Him happy, especially since we say we love Him and obedience shows Him that we do.

WHAT DOES THE BIBLE SAY?

Three Angel's Messages

• What is the first angel's message *(Rev. 14:6, 7)*?

• What does the first angel's message remind us of *(Ex. 31:16, 17)*?

• What is the second angel's message *(Rev. 14:8)*?

• Who is the Dragon, the Beast, and the false prophet *(Rev. 13:2–8)*?

• What is Babylon *(Rev. 16:19, 13)*?

✓ *DAILY WELLNESS CHECK*

__Am I still forgiving today?

__Am I being thankful today?

__Am I happy today?

__Am I helpful today?

__Am I obedient today?

__Did I eat more fruits and vegetables today?

__Was I intimate with God today?

__Am I ready for bed on time today?

__Did I drink enough water today?

__Did I overdo anything today?

__Did I exercise today?

__Am I taking deep breaths today?

__Did I get enough sunshine today?

__Did I dress appropriately today?

MY PRAYERS & CHALLENGES

....

....

....

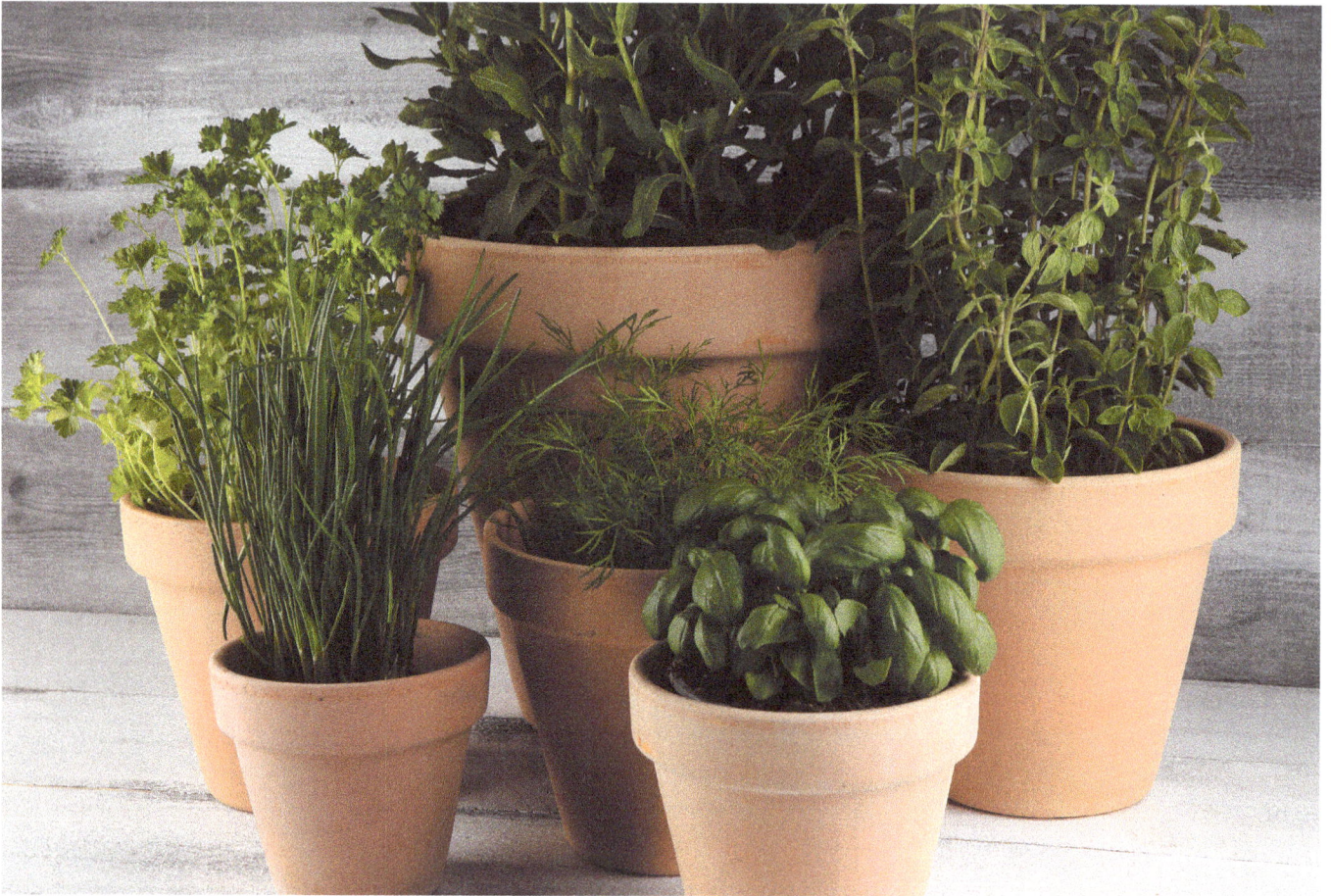

Physical Awareness

MORE HERBS AND HOW TO USE THEM IN COOKING (Hurd, Frank and Hurd, Rosalie. "A Good Cook…TEN TALENTS" 1968, pp. 164-166)

MINT (spearmint or peppermint): herb teas, sauces, honey, beverages, soups, applesauce, pie, salads, fruit, carrots, peas, cookies, frosting

ONION (bulb): salads, dressings, soups, vegetables, roasts, patties, bread, spaghetti sauces

OREGANO: pizza, tomatoes sauces, salads, meatless loaf

PAPRIKA (dry sweet pepper): salad dressing, coleslaw, red garnish, vegetables, potatoes

PARSLEY (flakes): soups, salads, tomatoes, vegetable dishes, potatoes, dressings, green garnish, brown rice

YOUR CHALLENGES ARE:

__to create your own special seasoning for gravies and veggie dishes.

__to do a **SECOND MILE ACT** for someone:

__to claim this promise: *"Bless the LORD, O my soul…Who redeemeth thy life from destruction, who crowneth thee with lovingkindness and tender mercies"* (Ps. 103:2, 4).

MENTAL & MORAL AWARENESS

GOD'S ROYAL LAW & COVENANT

Supplemental Reading: Exodus 20:1–17, Deuteronomy 4:13, James 2:8–12

#5 of God's 10 Commandments is about loving one another.

"Honour thy father and thy mother: that thy days may be long upon the land which the LORD thy God giveth thee" (Ex. 20:12).

WHAT DOES THE BIBLE SAY?

Three Angel's Messages

- What is the third angel's message *(Rev. 14:9–11)?*
- What is Babylon going to do *(Rev. 13:15–17)?*
- What will be the result to those who overcome the beast *(Rev. 15:2)?*
- Who gets the victory over the beast *(Rev. 14:12)?*

✓ *DAILY WELLNESS CHECK*

__*Am I still forgiving today?*

__*Am I being thankful today?*

__*Am I happy today?*

__*Am I helpful today?*

__*Am I obedient today?*

__*Did I eat more fruits and vegetables today?*

__*Was I intimate with God today?*

__*Am I ready for bed on time today?*

__*Did I drink enough water today?*

__*Did I overdo anything today?*

__*Did I exercise today?*

__*Am I taking deep breaths today?*

__*Did I get enough sunshine today?*

__*Did I dress appropriately today?*

MY PRAYERS & CHALLENGES

……

……

……

HEALTHY TIDBITS

Advantages of the two-meal plan:

- ◆ It stops children from nagging for snacks.
- ◆ It cuts down on the cost of food by ¼ to ⅓.
- ◆ It saves you an extra 30–90 minutes for special activities.
- ◆ It cuts kitchen chores by 30–60 minutes.
- ◆ It helps regulate body weight by improving metabolic efficiency.
- ◆ The burden is off the stomach in the evening, giving clarity of mind for evening study and worship.
- ◆ You can get into bed earlier and reap more of the early-to-bed benefits.
- ◆ Less sleep is needed because the digestive system is at rest.
- ◆ Blood is not drawn away from the skin, therefore the body can sleep better in a cooler room.
- ◆ In the morning, you will wake with a cleaner mouth and breath, clearer eyes, an alert mind, and no heavy bags under the eyes.
- ◆ The stomach is not exhausted but feels at peace.
- ◆ The body is more energetic and can work comfortably for hours before breakfast.
- ◆ Breakfast becomes a tasty delight.
- ◆ There is less temptation to snack between meals or eat an evening snack, both of which can sabotage a hearty breakfast.
- ◆ A clean and rested stomach produces healthy blood, which leads to better health.
- ◆ The stomach enjoys a longer period of rest, therefore, there is less danger of ulcers.
- ◆ Pregnant women who eat two meals have less trouble with morning sickness.
- ◆ Nursing mothers produce more milk.
- ◆ Be patient with the change. It takes a month or more to transition.

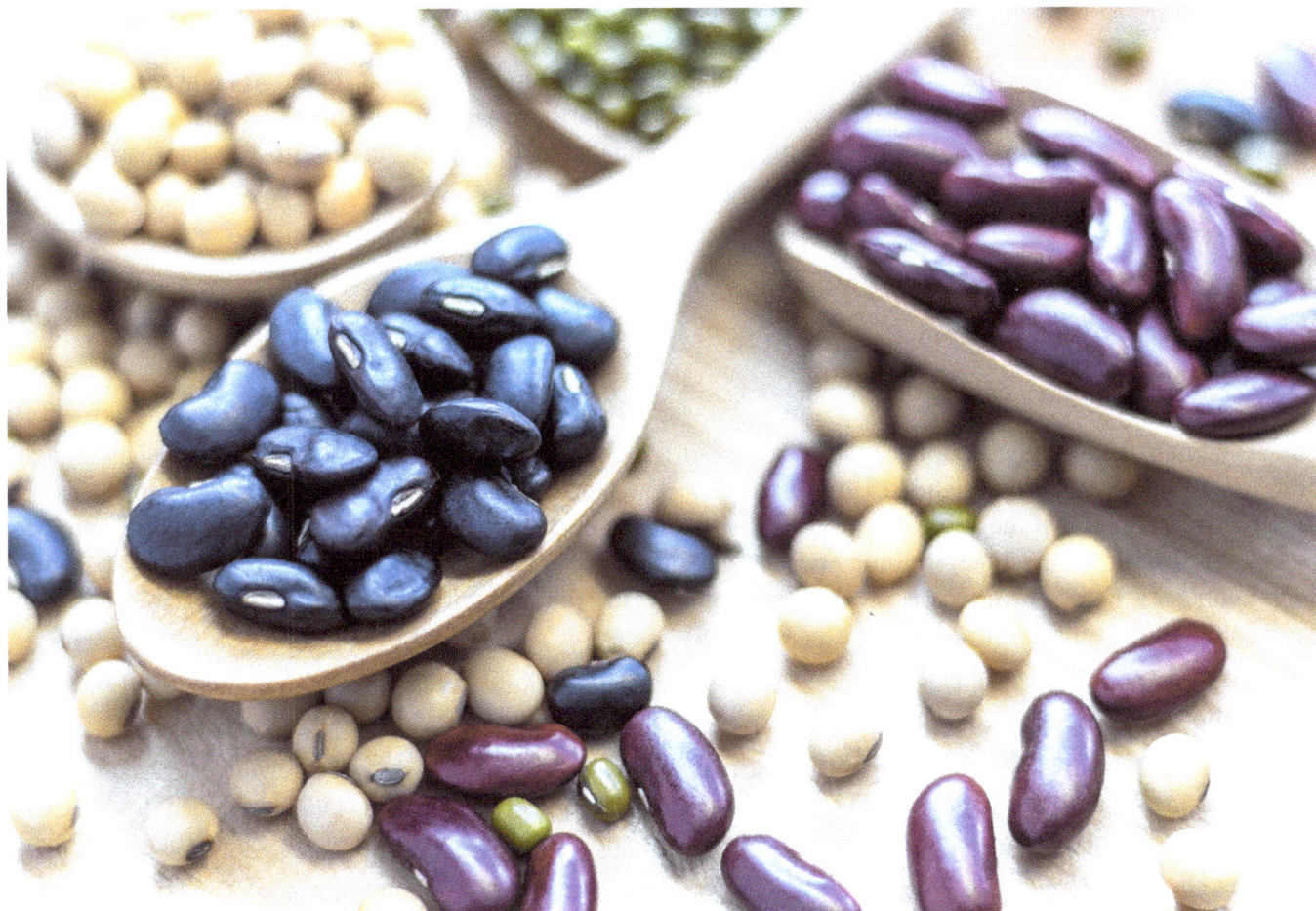

Physical Awareness

MORE ABOUT HEALTHY FOODS

Am I Getting Enough Protein?

One concern for many, is that they cannot get enough protein by eating only plant foods. You must consider this fact: animals get their protein from plants. It becomes recycled in animals. Why not get it from the same source as animals get it from? Plant sources of protein include nuts and legumes (beans).

Note: be careful how many nuts you are consuming in the form of nut butters.

A study shows that too much protein causes deterioration of kidney function, and is linked to increased risk of cancer (Zemel, et al. 1981, 2429-2433). **If the body is getting too much protein that it cannot properly metabolize, you will tend to have health problems, ranging from a strong body odor, joint pain, allergies, osteoporosis, heart disease, gout, cancer, earlier sexual maturity, decreased endurance, kidney stones, and kidney impairment. To eliminate this problem, drink more water and eat more fruits and vegetables.**

"Excessive protein intake has been linked to many health problems, from relatively benign and reversible conditions such as dehydration, constipation and nutritional deficiencies to obesity, heart and kidney diseases, insulin resistance diabetes, prostate cancer, decreased thyroid function, metabolic acidosis and reduced immune function" (Ogunjimi 2020).

What About Meat?

For ten generations before the flood, people who did not partake in eating flesh food had an average lifespan of 912 years. After the flood, there was no vegetation on the earth, so God gave humans permission to eat flesh food (see Gen. 9:3–5). However, the average lifespan of humans for 10 generations after the flood was 317 years, a decrease of 67%! God gave specific instructions regarding the eating of meat:

- Only clean animals are to be eaten (Lev. 11:1–20).
- Do not eat the blood (Gen. 9:4; Lev. 17:10–14).
- Do not eat the fat or the blood (Lev. 3:17).
- Eat it within three days of the animal being killed (Lev. 19:7).

The problem with eating flesh food is that it causes our life expectancy to decrease. We were not designed to eat flesh food. Our teeth were designed to grind, not tear. The amount of hydrochloric acid in our stomachs is not sufficient to break down the protein efficiently, or to kill the bacteria found in meat. Additionally, our mouths are alkaline, and our intestines are long and ridged. Carnivores have teeth that can tear the flesh, they have a higher concentration of hydrochloric acid in the stomach (ten times greater), their mouths are acidic, and they have a short, smooth intestines.

Purine is found in meats. This product can cause gout and kidney stones. Meat contains a lot of bacteria, which cannot be seen, smelled or tasted.

Leviticus 22:8 warns against eating any meat that has died of itself. You do not know what happened with the animal that you are eating unless you raised and killed it yourself. Pork, especially, contains parasites, like trichinosis. Pigs are scavengers; they eat refuse, decaying matter, and dung. Do you really want to be eating that?

Meat and fish contain a lot of cholesterol. Cholesterol is found only in animal products. The body can make its own, so it is not necessary for us to eat cholesterol.

What About Fish?

Fish is a source of protein that brings its own problems. There are many environmental concerns with eating fish since much of the water in which these fish swim has become polluted. Fish ingest large amounts of heavy metals, such as mercury, which is poisonous to the body. Babies have been born with central nervous system malformations and mental retardation as a result of mothers eating fish during pregnancy.

Flesh food increases the incidence of disease by ten times!

Meat Substitutes

Vegetarians who eat a lot of meat substitutes are also at risk for disease, as a result of a high protein diet with often high salt content. Read all labels.

Avoid mushrooms. They do not have any roots. There are fungi, growing from dead and decaying things.

Avoid fermented foods, such as vinegar, which irritates the stomach and rots your food.

YOUR CHALLENGES ARE:

__to eat a meatless meal.

__to eat a fishless meal.

__to carefully read labels on all meat substitutes.

__to do a **SECOND MILE ACT** for someone:

__**to claim this promise:** *"Whether therefore ye eat, or drink, or whatsoever ye do, do all to the glory of God"* (1 Cor. 10:31).

RECIPE FOR THE DAY

CHICKPEA A LA KING

½ cup. chopped onions

2 Tbsp. oil

2 Tbsp. water

3 cups water/garbanzo liquid

½ cup cashew pieces

4 tsp. sesame seeds

3 Tbsp. country-style seasoning

¼ tsp. salt

¾ tsp. garlic powder

1 Tbsp. onion powder

1 Tbsp. cornstarch

2 cups frozen green peas

½ cup chopped pimentos

2 cups cooked garbanzos (If salt free, add ¼ tsp. salt.)

SAUTE first 4 ingredients. Set aside. Blend next 8 ingredients on high 1–2 minutes or until thickened. Rinse peas with hot water for 10–15 seconds. Add onions, peas, and remaining ingredients to saucepan. Cook and stir for 2 more minutes. Serve over brown rice, flat noodles, or toast.

MENTAL & MORAL AWARENESS

GOD'S ROYAL LAW & COVENANT

Supplemental Reading: Exodus 20:1–17, Deuteronomy 4:13, James 2:8–12

#6 of God's Ten Commandments is about loving each other

"Thou shalt not kill" (Ex. 20:13).

WHAT DOES THE BIBLE SAY?

The True Church

- What is the church likened to *(Jer. 6:2)?*
- Who is the pure woman *(Rev. 12:1–6)?*
- What is the description of the bad woman *(Rev. 17:3–6)?*
- What happened to the pure woman *(Rev. 12:6, 14)?*
- Who is the child/man *(Rev. 12:4, 7)?*

✓ *DAILY WELLNESS CHECK*

__*Am I still forgiving today?*

__*Am I being thankful today?*

__*Am I happy today?*

__*Am I helpful today?*

__*Am I obedient today?*

__*Did I eat more fruits and vegetables today?*

__*Was I intimate with God today?*

__*Am I ready for bed on time today?*

__*Did I drink enough water today?*

__*Did I overdo anything today?*

__*Did I exercise today?*

__*Am I taking deep breaths today?*

__*Did I get enough sunshine today?*

__*Did I dress appropriately today?*

MY PRAYERS & CHALLENGES

....

....

....

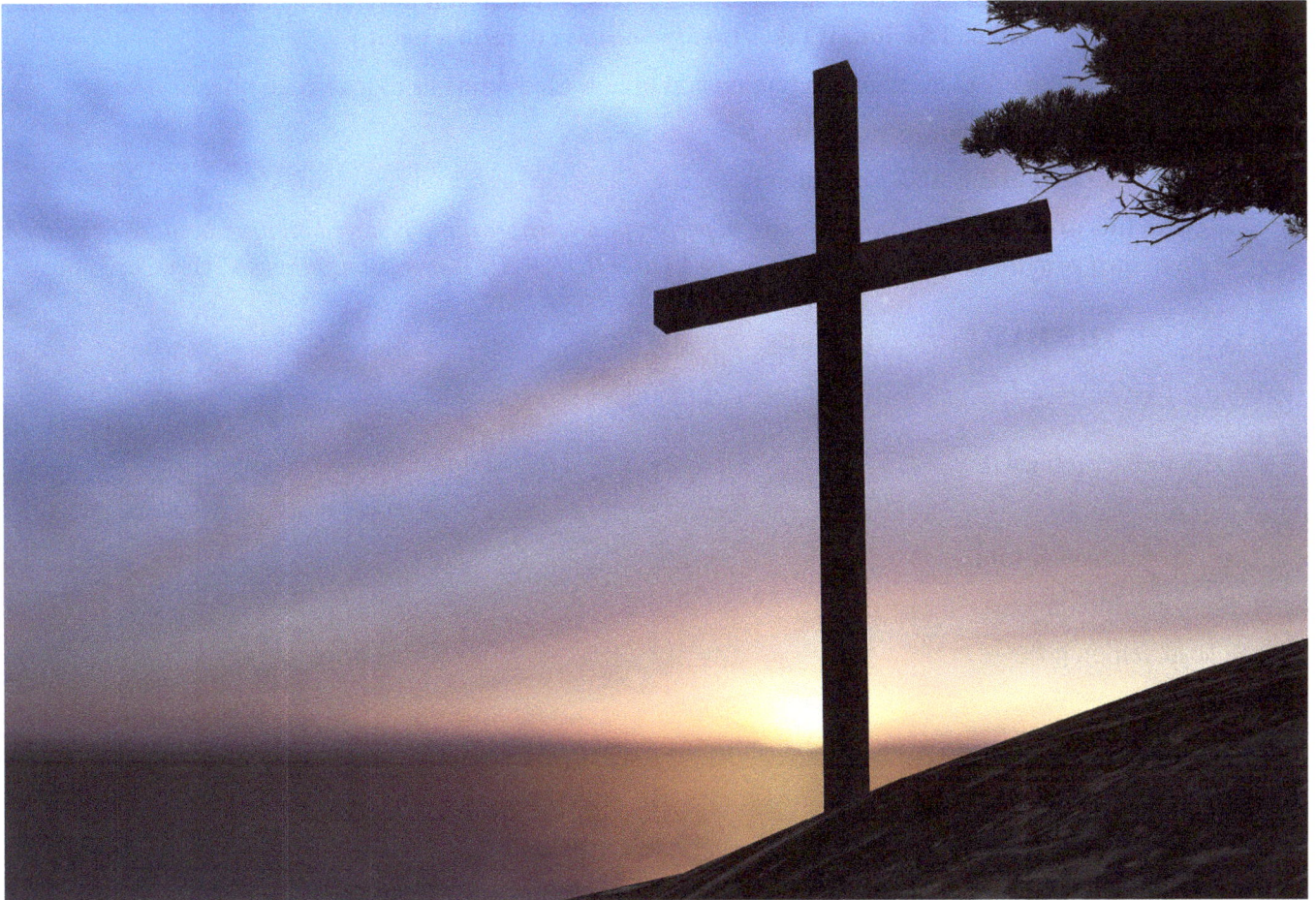

Physical Awareness

MORE ABOUT INTIMACY WITH GOD

Know that He is:

MERCIFUL

GRACIOUS

LONG-SUFFERING

ABUNDANT IN GOODNESS and TRUTH

KEEPING MERCY FOR THOUSANDS

FORGIVING OF INIQUITY, TRANSGRESSION and SIN

SLOW TO ANGER

OF GREAT KINDNESS

(see Exodus 34:6; Jonah 4:2; Micah 7:18)

YOUR CHALLENGES ARE:

__To start reading the Bible through (if you have not already started).

- ◆ **Start with the book of John.**
- ◆ **Read a chapter a day. These twenty-one chapters will help you develop the habit of spending time with your Lord and Savior. (It takes twenty-one days to form a habit.)**

__to read 1 Corinthians 13 every day to remind you of how God wants us to love each other.

__to memorize 1 Corinthian 13 and Psalms 91.

__to do a **SECOND MILE ACT** for someone:

__**to claim this promise:** *"Thou will keep him in perfect peace, whose mind is stayed on thee: because he trusteth in thee. Trust ye in the LORD for ever: for in the LORD JEHOVAH is everlasting strength"* (Isa. 26: 3, 4).

RECIPE FOR THE DAY

MAYONNAISE

1½ tsp. unflavored gelatin

¼ cup cold water

1 cup raw cashew or tofu

1 Tbsp. nutritional yeast

1½ Tbsp. lemon juice

1½ Tbsp. onion powder

1½ tsp. salt

¼ tsp. garlic powder

½ tsp. coriander (optional)

LET gelatin and water sit in blender for 5 minutes, then blend in other ingredients thoroughly.

MENTAL & MORAL AWARENESS

GOD'S ROYAL LAW & COVENANT

Supplemental Reading: Exodus 20:1–17, Deuteronomy 4:13, James 2:8–12

#7 of God's 10 Commandments is about not sleeping with someone other than your spouse.

"Thou shalt not commit adultery" (Ex. 20:14).

WHAT DOES THE BIBLE SAY?

The True Church

- • What is the special work of the true church *(Rev. 12:17)*?
- • What did Jesus say about His coming *(Rev. 22:7, 12)*?
- • Who is going to eat of the tree of life and live eternally *(Rev. 22:14)*?
- • What is God saying to you and me today *(Rev. 18:4)*?

✓ *DAILY WELLNESS CHECK*

__*Am I still forgiving today?*

__*Am I being thankful today?*

__*Am I happy today?*

__*Am I helpful today?*

__*Am I obedient today?*

__*Did I eat more fruits and vegetables today?*

__*Was I intimate with God today?*

__*Am I ready for bed on time today?*

__*Did I drink enough water today?*

__*Did I overdo anything today?*

__*Did I exercise today?*

__*Am I taking deep breaths today?*

__*Did I get enough sunshine today?*

__*Did I dress appropriately today?*

MY PRAYERS & CHALLENGES

....

....

....

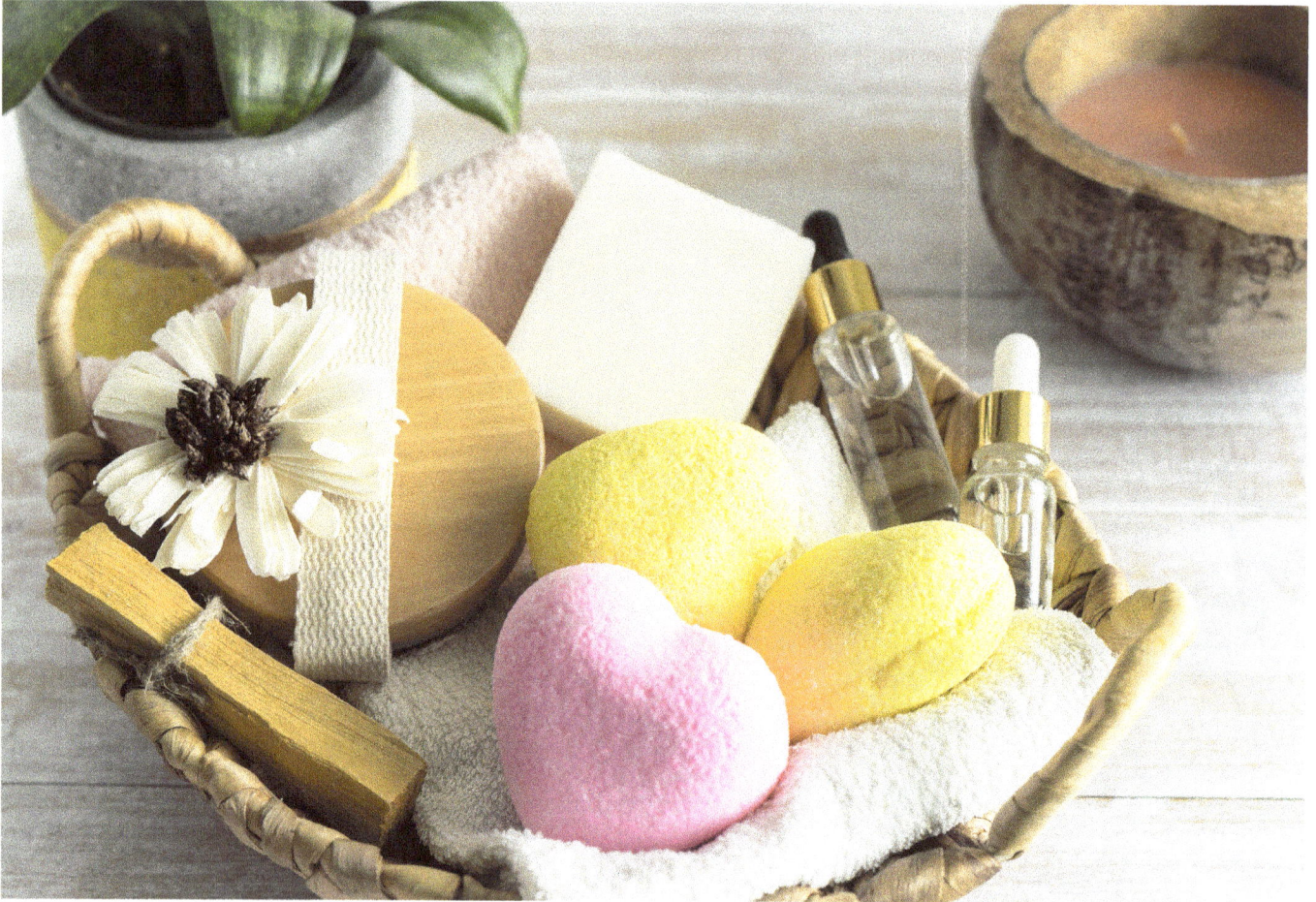

Physical Awareness

MORE FACTS ABOUT SLEEP

- Sleep reduces stress.
- Lack of sleep causes depression and contributes to physical, mental, and emotional trauma.
- Going to bed early helps the mind to organize information so that you can retrieve it easily.

YOUR CHALLENGES ARE:

__to keep your sleeping room dark and quiet.

__to take a warm bath to sooth and relax the nerves.

__to pray before bed. Ask your Heavenly Father to free your mind of concerns and to give you peace at night.

__to do a **SECOND MILE ACT** for someone:

__**to claim this promise:** *"My grace is sufficient for thee"* (2 Cor. 12:9).

RECIPE FOR THE DAY

SALSA

¼ cup red, yellow, or orange bell pepper

¼ cup green onion (scallions)

1 small onion

2 cloves garlic

8 fresh sprigs of cilantro

3 medium tomatoes

¼ cup (more or less) lime juice

1½ tsp. salt

2 tsp. onion powder

1 tsp. garlic powder

1 Tbsp. (or more) cayenne pepper

COMBINE the first 5 ingredients and blend until they are all finely chopped; then pour it into a bowl. Blend tomatoes separately until they turn into a sauce. Pour tomato sauce over vegetables, along with the remaining ingredients (seasoning), and mix together. Place in refrigerator to marinate for 1 hour.

MENTAL & MORAL AWARENESS

GOD'S ROYAL LAW & COVENANT

Supplemental Reading: Exodus 20:1–17, Deuteronomy 4:13, James 2:8–12

#8 of God's 10 Commandments says not to take what is not yours.

"Thou shalt not steal" (Ex. 20:15).

WHAT DOES THE BIBLE SAY?

Spirit of Prophecy

- What is the true church going to have *(Rev. 12:17)*?
- What is the testimony of Jesus *(Rev. 19:10)*?
- Whom does God use *(2 Peter 1:21)*?
- What happens when a prophet has a vision *(Ps. 89:19)*?

✓ *DAILY WELLNESS CHECK*

__*Am I still forgiving today?*

__*Am I being thankful today?*

__*Am I happy today?*

__*Am I helpful today?*

__*Am I obedient today?*

__*Did I eat more fruits and vegetables today?*

__*Was I intimate with God today?*

__*Am I ready for bed on time today?*

__*Did I drink enough water today?*

__*Did I overdo anything today?*

__*Did I exercise today?*

__*Am I taking deep breaths today?*

__*Did I get enough sunshine today?*

__*Did I dress appropriately today?*

MY PRAYERS & CHALLENGES

....

....

....

HEALTHY TIDBITS

COOKING BEANS TO IMPROVE DIGESTION

Wash beans thoroughly. Soak overnight or for eight hours. Rinse, drain, and freeze. This will break up the troublesome starch molecules, which cause gas and bloating. The next day, take frozen beans and boil in an uncovered pot for about ten minutes. Drain water and boil in new water until done.

While cooking, add a pinch of ginger or fennel. These will further remove more of the potential gas that causes bloating. Cook beans until soft. Add the salt near the end; it tends to slow down the cooking. Add the other spices and onions at the beginning of cooking. You can add a little coconut oil also. (Do not add any tomato items until beans are done because they will stop or slow the cooking process.)

If you want to sprout your beans to get ten to three hundred percent more nutrition from them, drain out all the water and put them in a large strainer-type colander. Cover with a cover that has holes like a flat strainer. Sit them on a plate to catch the extra water that drains off of them for one to two days. Wet them twice a day. If they are not too old, you will start to see the little sprouts. Then you can freeze them and proceed as directed above. A surprisingly sweet smell will be emanating from them.

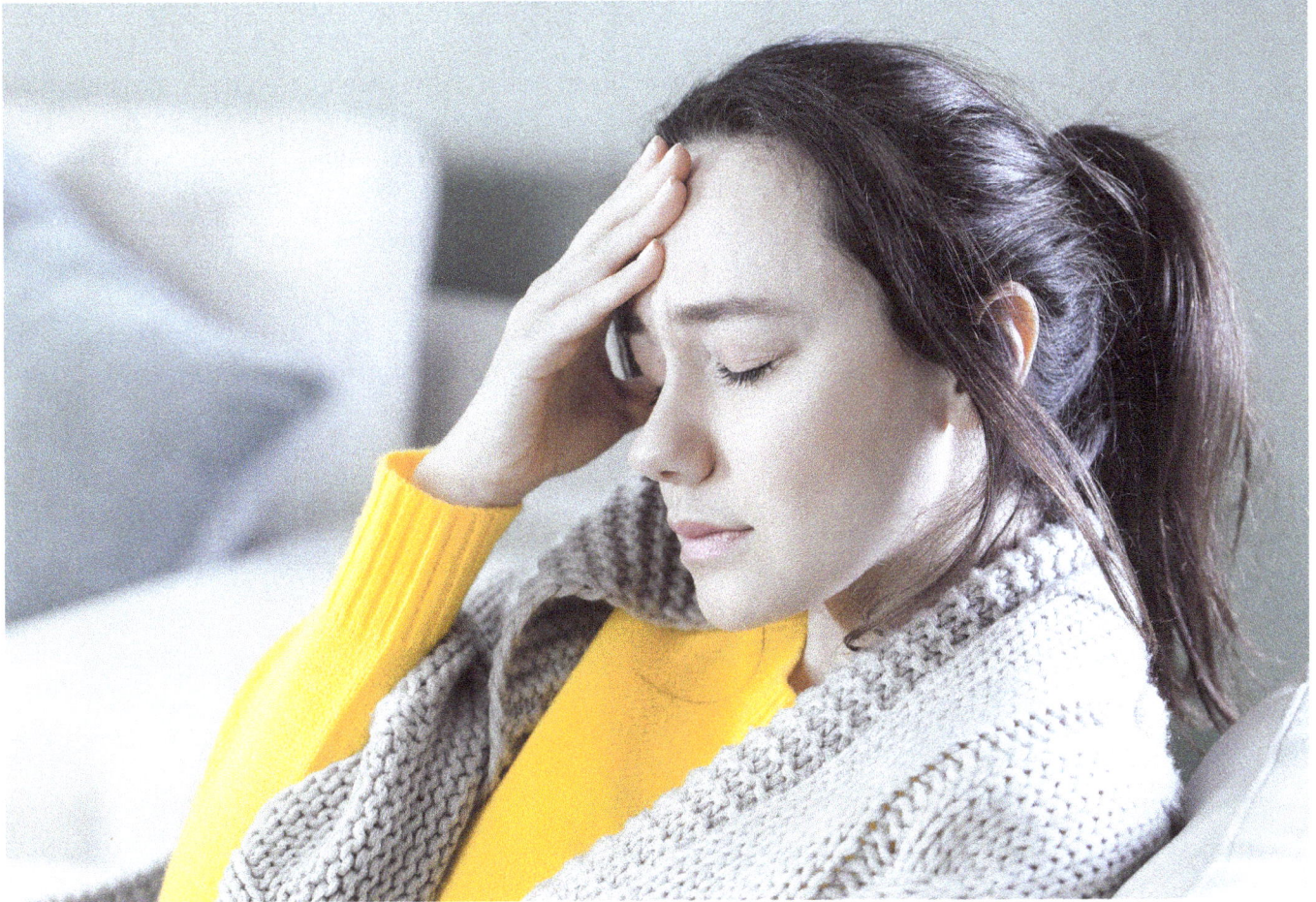

Physical Awareness

MORE FACTS ABOUT WATER

- Water is an appetite suppressant, so it helps you lose weight by reducing hunger.
- It quickly washes away the by-products of fat breakdown.
- Water has zero calories and it speeds up your metabolism, helping with weight loss.
- It helps relieve headaches and fatigue.
- Water helps you look younger by creating healthier skin.
- It improves memory since the brain is eighty-five percent water.
- Water helps you regulate body temperature, so it increases exercise endurance.
- Water helps create a positive attitude and mood.
- The lack of water makes you feel tired, depressed, confused, tense, and angry.

YOUR CHALLENGES ARE:

__to take a hot and cold shower

How To Benefit From Hot And Cold Showers

Hot and cold showers can prevent illnesses. With the hot and cold action, the immune system is built up and is stronger to fight diseases.

Take your shower or bath in water, as warm as you can take it. After cleaning yourself, washing off all the soap, turn all the hot water off, and turn the cold water all the way on for thirty seconds. Let the cold water hit all surfaces of your skin. Make sure that the cold water hits the back of your neck. The number of white blood cells (disease fighters) in the blood will increase greatly.

You may have to scream or do a cold dance in the shower. This cycle should be done at least once on a daily basis, but it can be repeated three times to fight off pain or the flu.

__to do a **SECOND MILE ACT** for someone:

__**claim this promise:** *"To him that is afflicted pity should be shewed from his friend"* (Job 6:14).

RECIPE FOR THE DAY

WHITE SAUCE

4 cups hot water

1 cup raw cashews

4 tsp onion powder

1 tsp. salt

1 Tbsp. chickenish seasoning

¼ cup cornstarch

BLEND until smooth. Next, cook over medium heat, stirring constantly until thick.

MENTAL & MORAL AWARENESS

GOD'S ROYAL LAW & COVENANT

Supplemental Reading: Exodus 20:1–17, Deuteronomy 4:13, James 2:8–12

#9 of God's Commandments means not to say untrue things about anyone.

"Thou shalt not bear false witness against thy neighbour" (Ex. 20:16).

WHAT DOES THE BIBLE SAY?

Spirit of Prophecy

- How can you know a true prophet *(Isa. 8:20)?*
- What is the fruit of a prophet *(Matt. 7:20)?*
- Does prophecy always come true *(Jer. 28:9)?*
- What are the gifts for *(Eph. 4:4–15)?*
- Do we have a prophet in the last days *(1 Cor. 1:4–8)?*

✓ *DAILY WELLNESS CHECK*

__*Am I still forgiving today?*

__*Am I being thankful today?*

__*Am I happy today?*

__*Am I helpful today?*

__*Am I obedient today?*

__*Did I eat more fruits and vegetables today?*

__*Was I intimate with God today?*

__*Am I ready for bed on time today?*

__*Did I drink enough water today?*

__*Did I overdo anything today?*

__*Did I exercise today?*

__*Am I taking deep breaths today?*

__*Did I get enough sunshine today?*

__*Did I dress appropriately today?*

MY PRAYERS & CHALLENGES

....

....

....

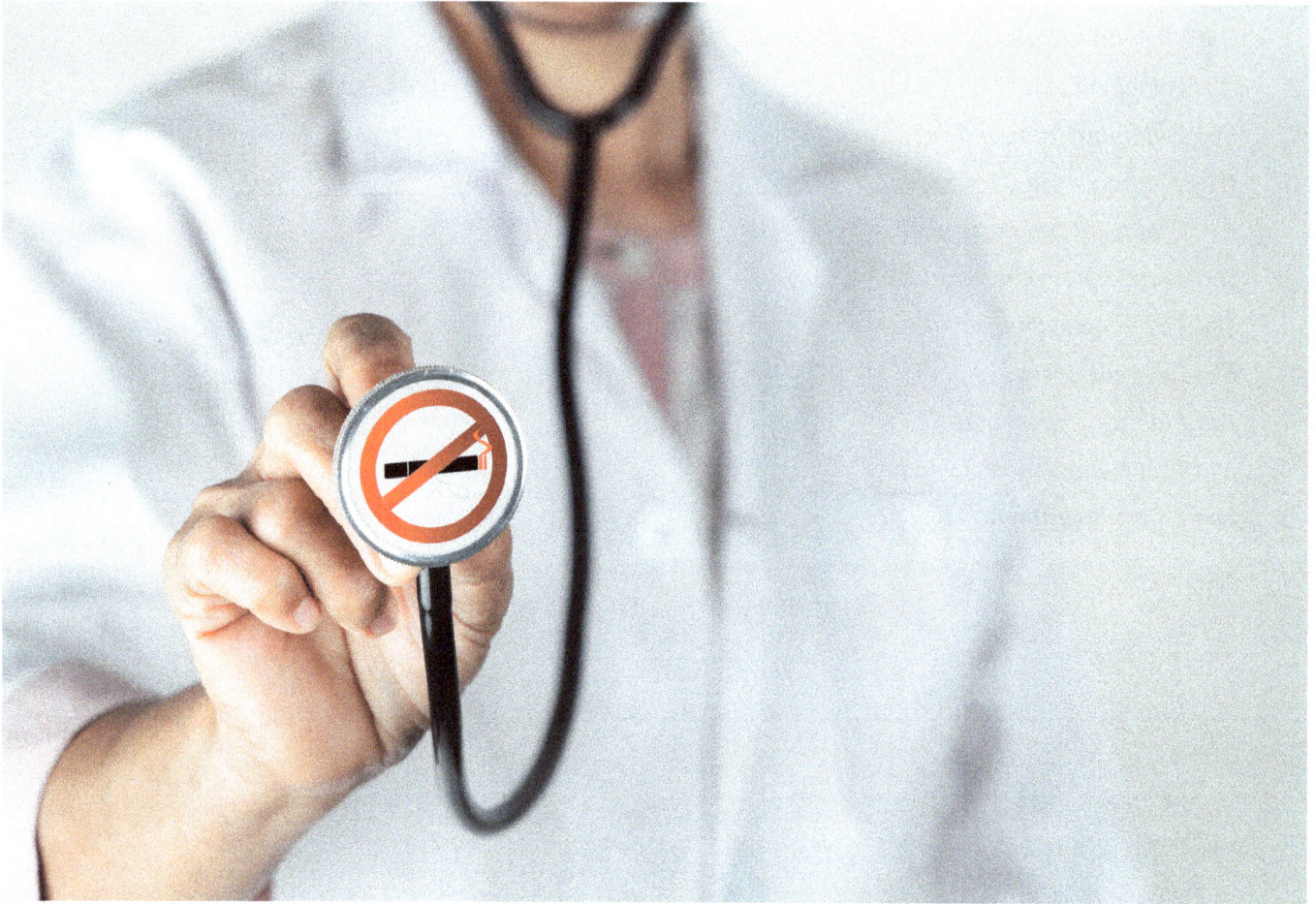

Physical Awareness

MORE ABOUT TEMPERANCE ALWAYS

ALCOHOL—is a known brain and intestinal toxin, and there is no safe level to drink when it comes to preventing cancer. It impairs reason, conscience, and judgement.

COFFEE—and some teas contain caffeine, which will increase heart palpitations, increase stress hormone levels, elevate blood sugar, and make sleep difficult.

TOBACCO—Smokers consume more coffee, alcohol and harmful drugs than nonsmokers. They also use more antibiotics, pain killers, sedatives, tranquilizers and sleeping pills than nonsmokers. (**See Day 40 for principles on how to quit.**)

DAMAGING DRUGS—destroy the central nervous system. They tear the entire body apart, starting with the nerves. The artificial high caused by the drug will lead to depression when the drug wears off.

YOUR CHALLENGES ARE:

__to give up two or more of the above issues.

__to do a **SECOND MILE ACT** for someone:

__**to claim this promise:** *"Bless the LORD, O my soul, and forget not all his benefits: Who forgiveth all thine iniquities; who healeth all thy diseases"* (Ps. 103:2, 3).

RECIPE FOR THE DAY

SPAGHETTI SAUCE

½ cup olive oil

1 medium onion, diced

2 medium/large carrots, diced

2 celery stalks, diced

6 cups tomato sauce

1 Tbsp. dried basil

½ clove garlic, minced

2 Tbsp. lemon juice

1 tsp. salt

SAUTE first 4 ingredients, then, add the rest. Simmer over low heat for 30 minutes.

MENTAL & MORAL AWARENESS

MORE FACTS ABOUT FORGIVENESS

Don't fool yourself; it hurts! Here is how you can change your heart:

- Admit to what hurts you and why it hurts. All this can be done in a conversation with God (praying).
- Talk about what the hurting is doing to you. Plead with the Lord for release from the pain.
- If another person hurts you, place yourself in their shoes, and think of what could have caused him or her to hurt you.
- Think of ways in which your experience has made you stronger, and how you can help others in similar situations.
- Reflect on God's mercy towards you. Anger and unforgiveness will burn you out and age you prematurely, so relax!

Mark Twain's famous quote says it best: "Anger is an acid that can do more harm to the vessel in which it is stored than to anything on which it is poured."

WHAT DOES THE BIBLE SAY?

Tithing

- Who owns everything *(Ps. 24:1)?*
- Who gave us power to be rich *(Deut. 8:18)?*
- What is tithe *(Lev. 27:32, 33)?*

- Who receives the tithe *(Num. 18:21)?*
- Does this apply to the New Testament *(1 Cor. 9:11–14)?*

✓ *DAILY WELLNESS CHECK*

__Am I still forgiving today?

__Am I being thankful today?

__Am I happy today?

__Am I helpful today?

__Am I obedient today?

__Did I eat more fruits and vegetables today?

__Was I intimate with God today?

__Am I ready for bed on time today?

__Did I drink enough water today?

__Did I overdo anything today?

__Did I exercise today?

__Am I taking deep breaths today?

__Did I get enough sunshine today?

__Did I dress appropriately today?

MY PRAYERS & CHALLENGES

....

....

....

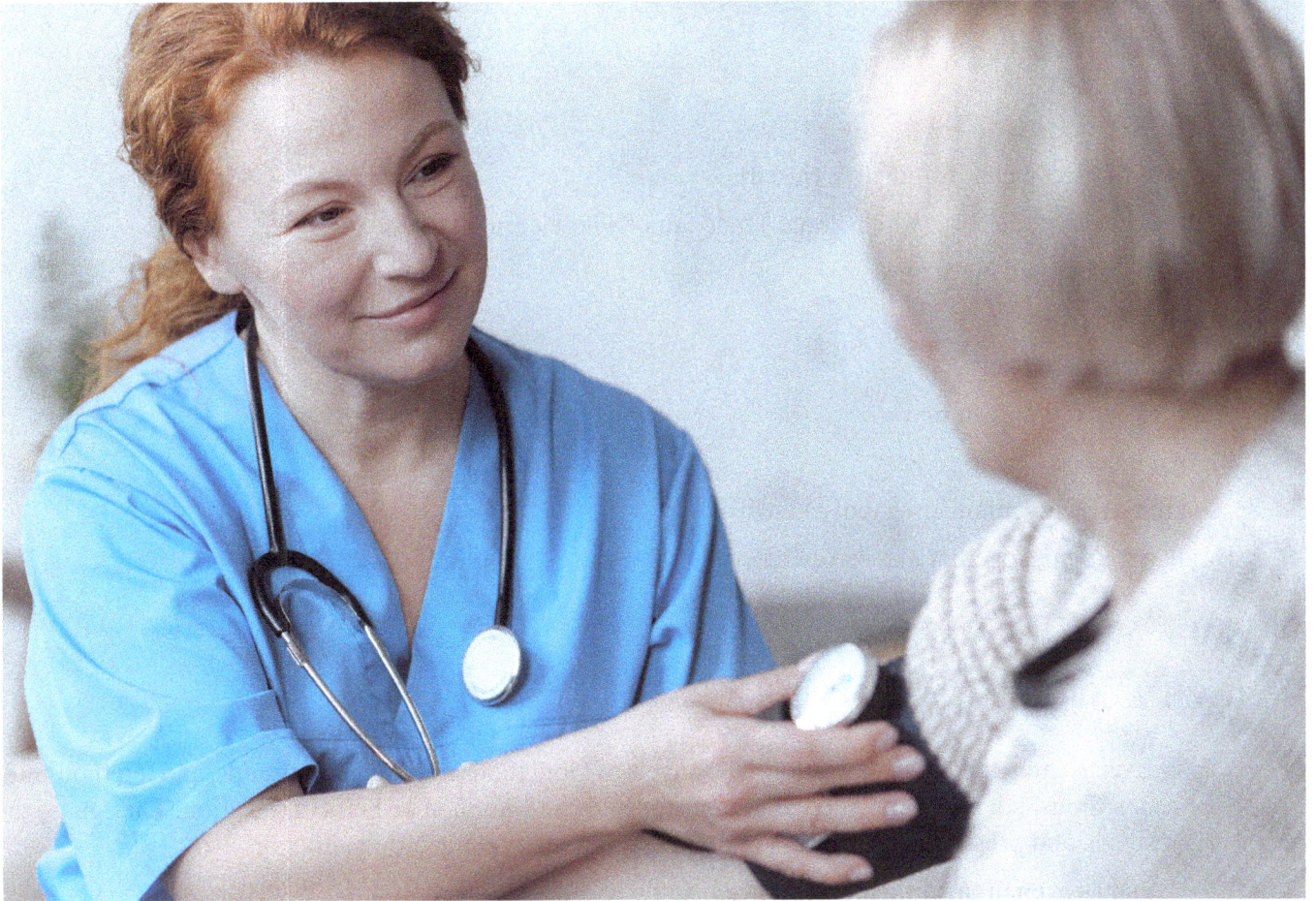

Physical Awareness

MORE FACTS ABOUT EXERCISING DAILY

- It regulates and lowers blood pressure.
- It helps bring the body to its ideal weight.
- It lowers the risk of cardiovascular disease.
- It increases strength and endurance.
- Physical and sweaty work is healthy exercise. It was the Creator's way to keep us strong.

Studies show that inactivity will increase the rate of degenerative diseases and conditions, such as heart disease, cancer, osteoporosis, anxiety, and depression.

YOUR CHALLENGES ARE:

__to find two friends to walk with you. (Having two exercise buddies ensures more accountability.)

__to find a safe place to walk (ex: mall, living room, hallway, well-lit outdoor area, or around the outside of the house).

__to do a **SECOND MILE ACT** for someone:

__**to claim this promise:** *"Beloved, I wish above all things that thou mayest prosper and be in health even as thy soul prospereth"* (3 John 2).

RECIPE FOR THE DAY

BLACK BEAN SALAD

1 or 2 cans of black beans (drained & rinsed)

1 small package frozen corn (whole kernel) or 1 can of whole corn, drained

1 can (small) chopped black olives

1 chopped red pepper

1 chopped green pepper

1 or 2 cups cooked, brown rice

Juice of 1 lime

Season to taste with cumin, oregano, cilantro

MIX all ingredients together and serve chilled.

MENTAL & MORAL AWARENESS

MORE FACTS ABOUT THANKFULNESS

- All heaven is interested in our salvation. The angels of God, thousands upon thousands, and ten thousand times ten thousand, are commissioned to minister to those who shall be heirs of salvation. They guard us against evil, and press back the powers of darkness that are seeking our destruction.
- Give thanks even in the difficult moments.
- Songs are weapons that we can always use against discouragement.
- Praise and thanksgiving should be expressed in song, especially when tempted. Do not voice your feelings; just sing in faith and thanksgiving to God.
- As you open your heart to the sunlight of the Savior's presence, you shall receive health and His blessings.

WHAT DOES THE BIBLE SAY?

Tithing

- What is the reason for paying tithe *(1 Sam. 15:22)?*
- What is the promise for those who are faithful in paying tithe *(Matt. 3:8–11)?*
- What can we give besides tithes *(Ps. 96:8)?*
- Who does God love *(2 Cor. 9:7)?*

✓ *DAILY WELLNESS CHECK*

__*Am I still forgiving today?*

__*Am I being thankful today?*

__*Am I happy today?*

__*Am I helpful today?*

__*Am I obedient today?*

__*Did I eat more fruits and vegetables today?*

__*Was I intimate with God today?*

__*Am I ready for bed on time today?*

__*Did I drink enough water today?*

__*Did I overdo anything today?*

__*Did I exercise today?*

__*Am I taking deep breaths today?*

__*Did I get enough sunshine today?*

__*Did I dress appropriately today?*

MY PRAYERS & CHALLENGES

....

....

....

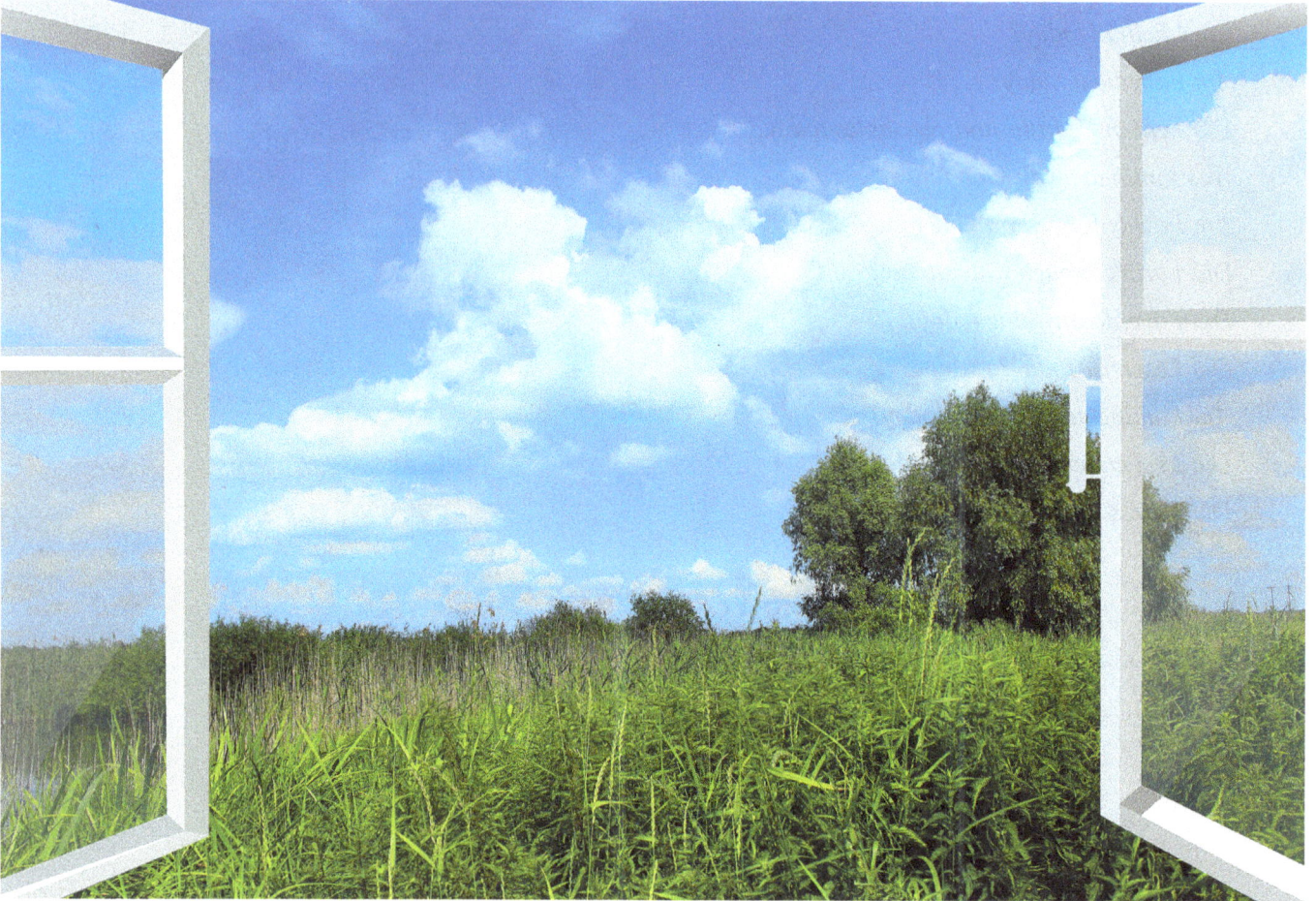

Physical Awareness

MORE FACTS ABOUT PURE, FRESH AIR

Oxygenated blood will keep you healthy. Here are some of the ways to get more oxygen into your body:

Ventilation: Open windows. Avoid car exhaust, tobacco smoke, and stuffy, ill-ventilated rooms.

Deep breathing: Take several deep breaths to clear the mind and increase the energy level. Consciously use your stomach muscles to fill and empty your lungs several times a day until deep breathing becomes a habit.

Exercise: Whenever possible, get good exercise outside in the morning when the air is cleaner.

Posture: Stand erect and walk tall so your lungs can breathe deeply, which will soon become a habit.

Clothing: Loose clothing allows the lungs freedom to inflate. Tight clothing restricts breathing.

Plants: They absorb carbon dioxide from the air and produce oxygen for us to breathe.

A rural environment: Fresh country air soothes the nerves, stimulates the appetite, and induces sound and refreshing sleep.

YOUR CHALLENGES ARE:

__to ventilate your home and car

__to make deep breathing a habit

__to exercise (whenever possible) outside in the morning

__to stand erect and walk tall

__to wear loose clothing

__to keep a plant or two in the house

__to visit the country often or move to the country

__to do a **SECOND MILE ACT** for someone:

__**to claim this promise:** *"Be strong and of a good courage; be not afraid, neither be thou dismayed: for the LORD they God is with thee whithersoever thou goest"* (Josh. 1:9).

RECIPE FOR THE DAY

GARLIC SPREAD

8–10 garlic cloves

2 cups olive oil

1 ½ tsp. salt

1 cup nutritional yeast flakes (optional)

½ cup fresh parsley, chopped; or 2 Tbsp. dried parsley

BLEND all ingredients. Brush spread onto bread slices. Sprinkle with parsley and bake in oven at 350 degrees for 5 minutes, or until golden.

MENTAL & MORAL AWARENESS

GOD'S ROYAL LAW & COVENANT

Supplemental Reading: Exodus 20:1–17, Deuteronomy 4:13, James 2:8–12

#10 of God's 10 Commandments is about not desiring another person's possessions.

"Thou shalt not covet they neighbour's house, thou shalt not covet thy neighbor's wife, nor his manservant, nor his maidservant, nor his ox, nor his ass, nor any thing that is thy neighbour's" (Ex. 20:17).

WHAT DOES THE BIBLE SAY?

Baptism

- Does God require Baptism *(Mark 16:16)?*
- What did Jesus do about Baptism *(Mark 1:9–11)?*
- Why was Jesus baptized *(1 Peter 2:21)?*
- What did Philip and the Eunuch do *(Acts 8:36–39)?*
- Why are we baptized *(Col. 2:12)?*
- Should we baptize people *(Matt. 28:19, 20)?*

✓ *DAILY WELLNESS CHECK*

__*Am I still forgiving today?*

__*Am I being thankful today?*

__*Am I happy today?*

__*Am I helpful today?*

__*Am I obedient today?*

__*Did I eat more fruits and vegetables today?*

__*Was I intimate with God today?*

__*Am I ready for bed on time today?*

__*Did I drink enough water today?*

__*Did I overdo anything today?*

__*Did I exercise today?*

__*Am I taking deep breaths today?*

__*Did I get enough sunshine today?*

__*Did I dress appropriately today?*

MY PRAYERS & CHALLENGES

....

....

....

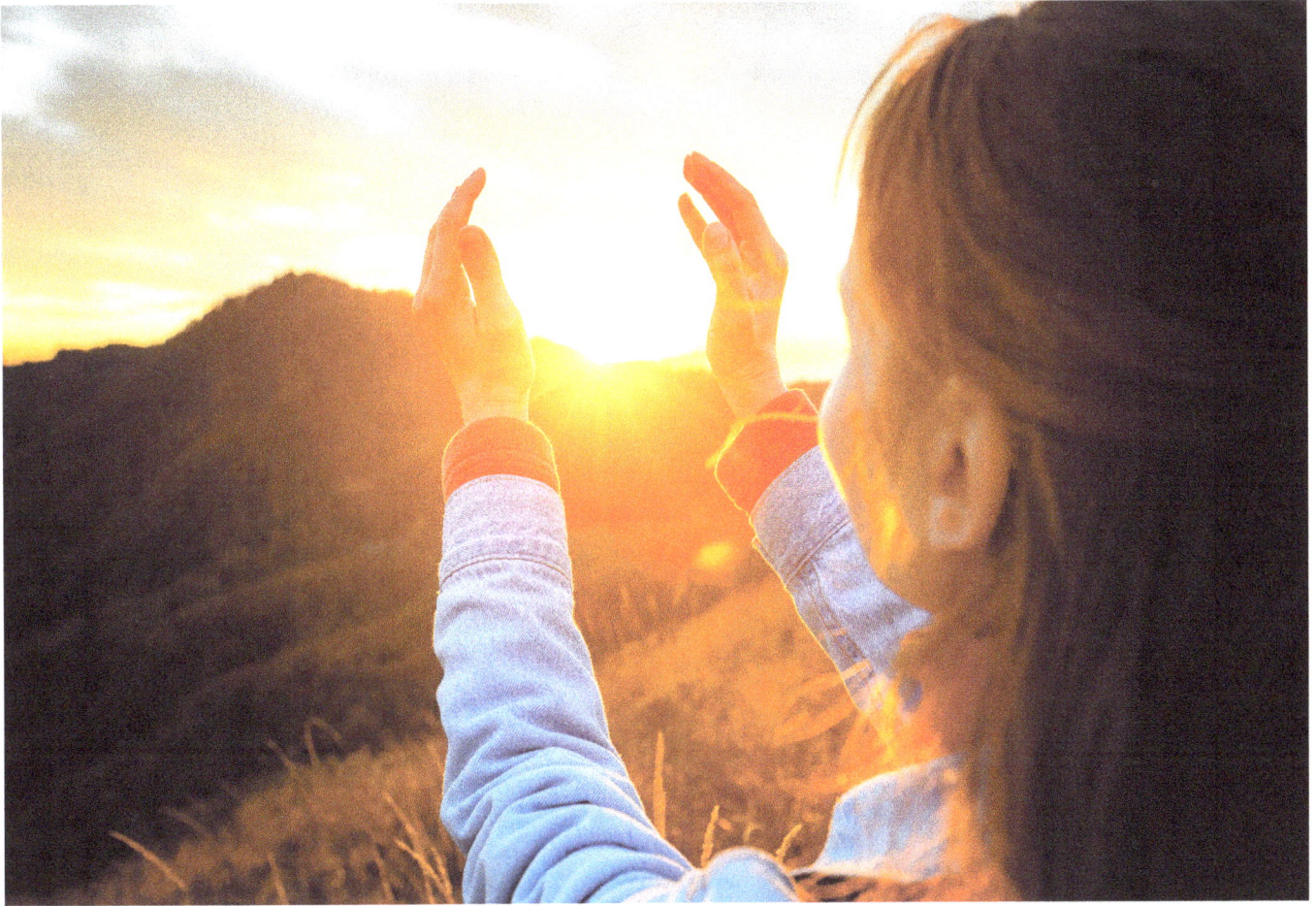

Physical Awareness

MORE FACTS ABOUT SUNLIGHT

- It increases the number of white blood cells and stimulates their ability to kill germs and cancer cells in our bodies.
- It builds up the immune system.
- It improves liver function and helps the body to eliminate toxic chemicals and pollutants.
- It is a good treatment for jaundice in newborn babies.
- It gives our body natural vitamin D and helps to lower cholesterol.
- It increases the amount of blood that is pumped into the heart.
- It helps stabilize blood sugar levels.
- It increases the volume of oxygen in the blood and improves circulation.

YOUR CHALLENGES ARE:

__to spend time outdoors every day while smiling, physically working, and rejoicing in song.

__to avoid wearing sunglasses, starting with 10 minutes a day. (Some sun is good for the eyes, but avoid looking directly at the sun. Just enjoy the warmth on your face)

__to do a **SECOND MILE ACT** for someone:

__**to claim this promise:** *"I perceive that there is nothing better, than that a man should rejoice in his own works; for that is his portion: for who shall bring him to see what shall be after him"* (Eccles. 3:22)?

RECIPE FOR THE DAY

PETE'S OAT BURGERS

Part 1:

2½ cups water

5 tsp. soy sauce or 2 tsp. salt

¼ cup oil

1 medium onion, chopped

½ tsp. Italian seasoning

2 tsp. onion powder

1 Tbsp. nutritional yeast (optional)

Part 2:

2 cups dry oatmeal

1 cup pecan, cashew, or sunflower meal

BOIL all the Part 1 ingredients for 2 minutes. Then add the Part 2 ingredients. MIX and let stand until cool or cold. Form patties by hand or use a hamburger press; place onto an oiled cookie sheet. Bake at 350 degrees to 20–30 minutes.

MENTAL & MORAL AWARENESS

MORE ABOUT LENDING A HELPING HAND

- The fifty-eighth chapter of Isaiah is a prescription for sickness of the body and of the soul. If we desire health and true joy, we must put these principles into practice.

- Good deeds are twice a blessing, benefiting both the giver and the receiver of the kindness. The consciousness of right-doing is one of the best medicines for diseased bodies and minds. Make it your aim to bless those around you, by finding ways to be helpful, both to the members of your own family and to others.

- Let the burden of your own weakness, sorrow, and pain be cast upon the compassionate Savior.

WHAT DOES THE BIBLE SAY?

Baptism

- What is rebaptism *(Acts 19:1–5)?*
- What is the memorial of the resurrection *(Rom. 6:3, 4)?*
- What does it mean to "put on Christ" *(Gal. 3:27)?*
- Should Christians be baptized *(1 John 2:6)?*
- What will happen if we follow Christ's command *(Rev. 22:14)?*

✓ *DAILY WELLNESS CHECK*

__*Am I still forgiving today?*

__*Am I being thankful today?*

__*Am I happy today?*

__*Am I helpful today?*

__*Am I obedient today?*

__*Did I eat more fruits and vegetables today?*

__*Was I intimate with God today?*

__*Am I ready for bed on time today?*

__*Did I drink enough water today?*

__*Did I overdo anything today?*

__*Did I exercise today?*

__*Am I taking deep breaths today?*

__*Did I get enough sunshine today?*

__*Did I dress appropriately today?*

MY PRAYERS & CHALLENGES

....

....

....

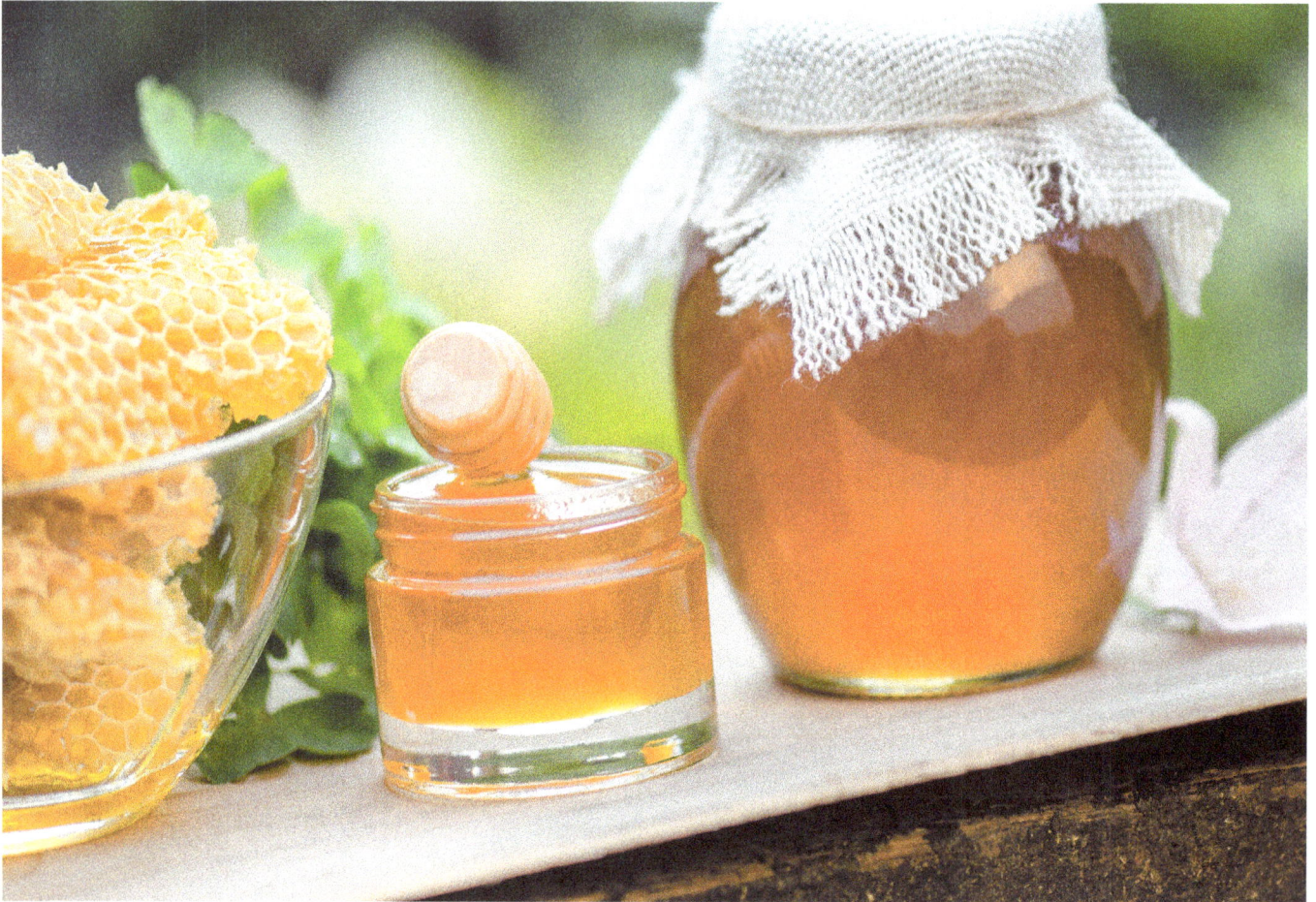

Physical Awareness

TAKING A CLOSER LOOK AT SUGAR

Sugar:

- Has empty calories, which means, no vitamins, minerals, or fiber, yet it requires these nutrients in order to be digested.

- Is a concentrated energy source void of fiber and causes you to overeat.

- Stops white blood cells from fighting infection and decreases resistance to disease.

- Increases dental decay.

- Quickly converts to fat (triglycerides) in the blood and increases the risk of obesity, heart disease, and diabetes.

YOUR CHALLENGE IS:

__to avoid candy or other sweets between meals.

__to avoid using sweets as a reward.

__to keep sugar off the table. Instead, keep raisins, dates, and other dried fruits on the table for natural sweeteners.

__to use concentrated sweeteners such as Sucanat, molasses, barley malt, honey, or date sugar.

__to develop a list of dessert recipes and cut the sweetener amount by a third or a half.

__to resist buying breakfast cereals where sugar is the first or second ingredient.

__to avoid desserts that use milk, sugar, and eggs together, since they can ferment when combined.

__to eat dessert in small portions after your dinner meal.

__to use unsweetened fruit juice rather than heavily sugared ones.

__to use fruit canned in its own juices rather than fruit canned in heavy syrup.

__to use apple juice concentrate as a sweetener.

__to do a **SECOND MILE ACT** for someone:

__**to claim this promise:** *"And the LORD hath [acknowledged] thee this day to be his peculiar people, as he hath promised thee, and that thou shouldest keep all his commandments"* (Deut. 26:18).

RECIPE FOR THE DAY

BAKED BEANS

6 cups cooked pinto or navy beans

½ cup water or bean broth

1 (16 oz.) can tomatoes

1 chopped onion

2 garlic cloves

¼ cup molasses

Salt to taste

MIX all ingredients together. Cook in a saucepan until onion is tender, or bake uncovered at 350 degrees for 60 minutes.

MENTAL & MORAL AWARENESS

FACTS ABOUT OBEYING WILLINGLY

- We must not withhold any service or means from God that we have made a pledge or covenant to fulfill.

- The purpose of all God's commandments is to reveal our duty, not only to God, but to our fellow humans.

- We rob our souls of rich blessings when our selfish hearts question or dispute the right of God to make requirements of us. Our selfish hearts usually convince us not to follow the requirements. Heart and mind and soul are to be merged in the will of God.

WHAT DOES THE BIBLE SAY?

Church Standards

- What principle should guide Christians at all times in their choice of reading, television, radio, and other forms of entertainment *(Phil. 4:8)?*
- What high standard does Peter point to regarding jewelry and fashion *(1 Peter 3:1–4)?*
- Should God be glorified in every aspect of a believer's life *(1 Cor. 10:31, 32)?*
- How did God regard immorality in Israel *(1 Cor. 10:6–8)?*
- Should two Christians go to court against each other *(1 Cor. 6:1–7)?*

✓ *DAILY WELLNESS CHECK*

__Am I still forgiving today?

__Am I being thankful today?

__Am I happy today?

__Am I helpful today?

__Am I obedient today?

__Did I eat more fruits and vegetables today?

__Was I intimate with God today?

__Am I ready for bed on time today?

__Did I drink enough water today?

__Did I overdo anything today?

__Did I exercise today?

__Am I taking deep breaths today?

__Did I get enough sunshine today?

__Did I dress appropriately today?

MY PRAYERS & CHALLENGES

....

....

....

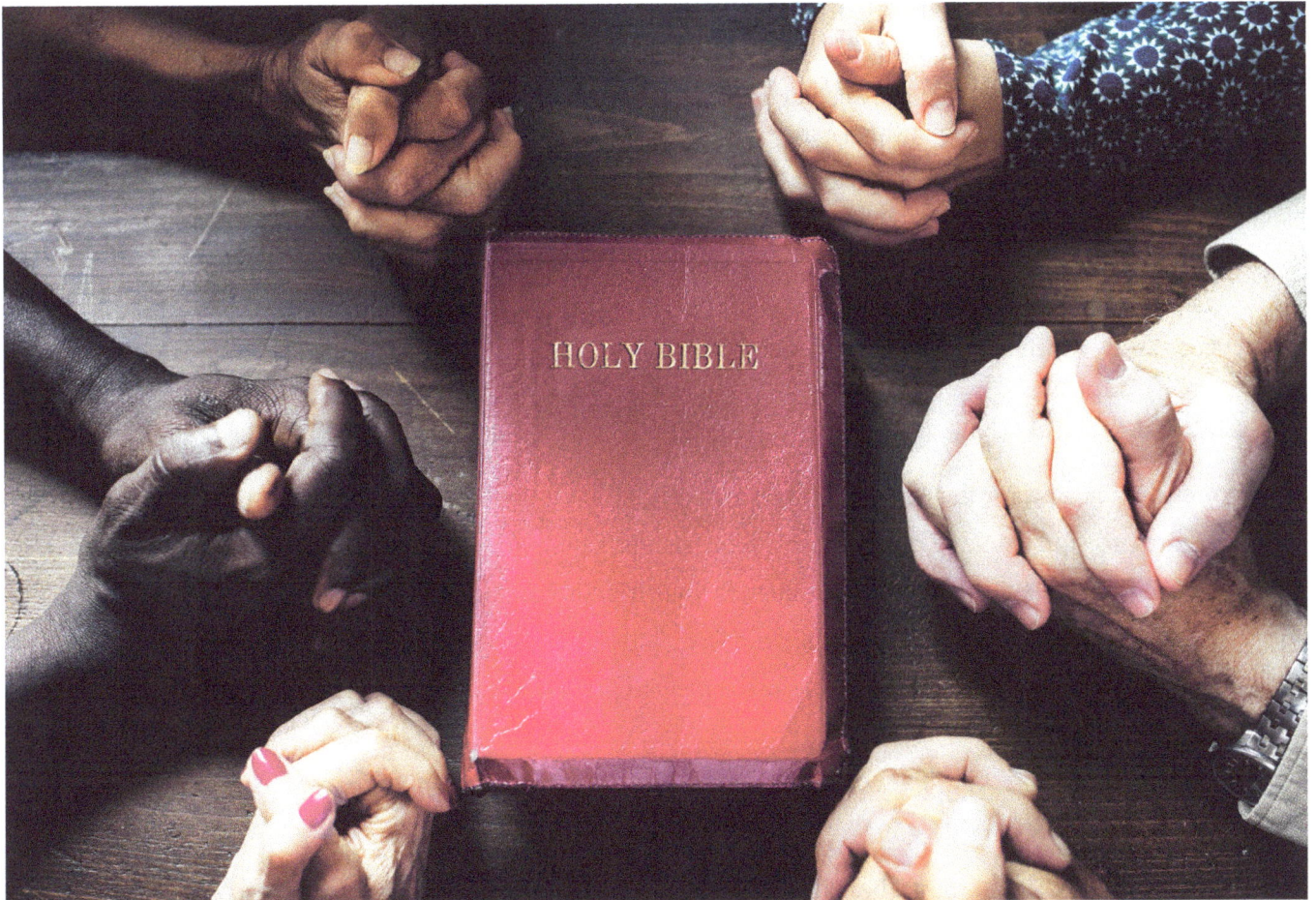

Physical Awareness

PRINCIPLES IN QUITTING SMOKING

1. First, make the decision not to smoke. Visualize it and verbalize it. Your brain will start releasing health-enhancing chemicals that aid in resisting cravings to smoke.

2. Trust that our heavenly Father will help you. All you need to do is ask and believe (see Matt. 7:7; Phil. 4:13).

3. Give yourself a **Salt Glow** treatment.

4. Bathe frequently in hot baths or showers to help remove toxins quickly.

5. Drink at least half your body weight in water; it will help flush out the nicotine.

6. Have a regular, daily routine for eating, drinking, exercising, sleeping, and other major activities. Stay on this program.

7. Do not sit around after you eat. Start a new routine. Take a 10–20 minute digestive walk. This will be great to keep your blood sugar normal.

8. Avoid stimulants. Caffeine and nicotine are stimulants and are cousins. "The use of tobacco encourages the appetite for liquor; and the use of tobacco and liquor invariably lessens nerve power" (White 1997, p. 109)

9. Avoid highly-spiced foods, fried foods, rich foods, and foods high in sugar. These things increase the craving for cigarettes.

10. Eat more fruits, whole grains, and vegetables. To get additional enzymes, include fresh fruit or vegetable juice in your diet as often as you can.

11. Whenever a craving comes, place one or two tablespoons of lemon juice in your mouth.

12. Take full deep breaths to relax you, to remove toxins, and to strengthen your lungs.

13. Make a cigarette out of a straw by cutting it to the length of a cigarette. Place a few drops of peppermint on a piece of cotton ball and stuff it into the straw. This is your new cigarette until the taste for a cigarette goes away, which should be about a week or two.

YOUR CHALLENGES ARE:

__to reward yourself for finishing the program.

__to share this stop-smoking program with your friends

__to share the 40-Day+ Wellness program with your friends and family

__to do a **SECOND MILE ACT** for someone:

__**to claim this promise:** *"Thy hands have made me and fashioned me: give me understanding, that I may learn thy commandments" (Ps. 119:73).*

HERBS AND HOW TO USE THEM IN COOKING (Hurd, Frank and Hurd, Rosalie. "A Good Cook… TEN TALENTS" 1968, pp. 164-166)

ROSEMARY—Soups, stews, roasts, boiled potatoes, peas, turnips, salad dressing

SAGE—Meatless loaf, patties, roasts, stuffing, butter (to reduce need for garlic), herbal tea, green salads, tofu

THYME—Soups, stews, stuffing, meatless dishes, fresh tomatoes, roasts, patties, carrots, beets

These seasonings are essential:

TURMERIC——Salad dressing, flavoring and coloring, sandwich spreads, scrambled tofu (soybean curd)

ITALIAN SEASONING—contains marjoram, rosemary, thyme, oregano, savory, and sage. (Great with onions in sautéed vegetables.)

*If cooking time is more than one hour, add herbs for just the last hour (retains more vitamins).

MENTAL & MORAL AWARENESS

Shall we be swept away by the strong tide of transgression and apostasy, or shall the righteous search the Scriptures and know for themselves the conclusions upon which the salvation of their souls depend? Those who make the Word of God their main counsel will esteem the law of God, and their appreciation for it will rise.

WHAT DOES THE BIBLE SAY?

Church Standards

• What should be our attitude towards divorce *(1 Cor. 7:10)?*

- How can a Christian avoid being worldly *(Rom. 12:1, 2)?*

- Is God concerned with the words we speak *(Eph. 5:3, 4)?*

- How should Christians relate to one another when differences arise? *(Eph. 4:22–32)?*

- What kind of people are preparing to meet Jesus when He comes a second time *(2 Peter 3:12–14)?*

✓ *DAILY WELLNESS CHECK*

__*Am I still forgiving today?*

__*Am I being thankful today?*

__*Am I happy today?*

__*Am I helpful today?*

__*Am I obedient today?*

__*Did I eat more fruits and vegetables today?*

__*Was I intimate with God today?*

__*Am I ready for bed on time today?*

__*Did I drink enough water today?*

__*Did I overdo anything today?*

__*Did I exercise today?*

__*Am I taking deep breaths today?*

__*Did I get enough sunshine today?*

__*Did I dress appropriately today?*

MY PRAYERS & CHALLENGES

. . . .

. . . .

. . . .

HEALTHY TIDBITS

A Lasting Miracle

We must keep the perspective of what we are to accomplish. Our goal is not just to follow the natural laws of health. They are important to help us keep our bodies clean, but our bodies are temporary. All of Christ's miracles were temporary: Lazarus died again, blind Bartimaeus had his eyes closed in death, and Peter never walked on water a second time.

Every one of Christ's miracles were temporary, **except one:** the miracle of salvation. The physical tools we have at our disposal are only important because they can bring people to a saving knowledge of Christ. If we lose sight of that fact, we have lost sight of the goal.

The message of wellness is that you do not have to be stuck where you are. You can come to God. When you cooperate with Him, He will open His storehouse and give you what you would not get otherwise. Even if our early length of life is not extended, a relationship will grow that makes this life more meaningful and prepares us for the next.

By keeping this in perspective we allow a restoration to the image of God in all facets, as with Joseph in Egypt. The Bible says Joseph was true to God, and God gave him favor in Potiphar's eyes: *"And the LORD was with Joseph, and he was a prosperous man; and he was in the house of his master the Egyptian. And Joseph found grace [favor] in his sight, and he served him: and he made him overseer of his house, and all that he had he put into his hand."* (Gen. 39:2, 4). We must share with our friends and family the blessings of healthy living.

We often attempt to live healthy lives simply for the present. We want to decrease pain, to add years to our lives, or to feel better about how we look. However, the supreme reason to live healthfully *should be* to live for the future reward of eternity "that fadeth not away" (1 Peter 5:4).

WHAT DOES THE BIBLE SAY?

State Of The Dead

- Who only is immortal *(1 Timothy 6:14-16)?*

- What lie did Satan tell *(Genesis 3:2-4)?*

- How did God make man *(Genesis 2:7)?*

- What do the dead know *(Ecclesiastes 9:5-10)?*

- What happens at death *(Psalms 146:4)?*

- Can the soul die *(Ezekiel 18:4)?*

- What did Jesus say about death *(John 11:11-14)?*

- When will the dead be raise *(I Thessalonians 4:16, 17)?*

- When do we receive immortality *(1 Corinthian 15:51-55)?*

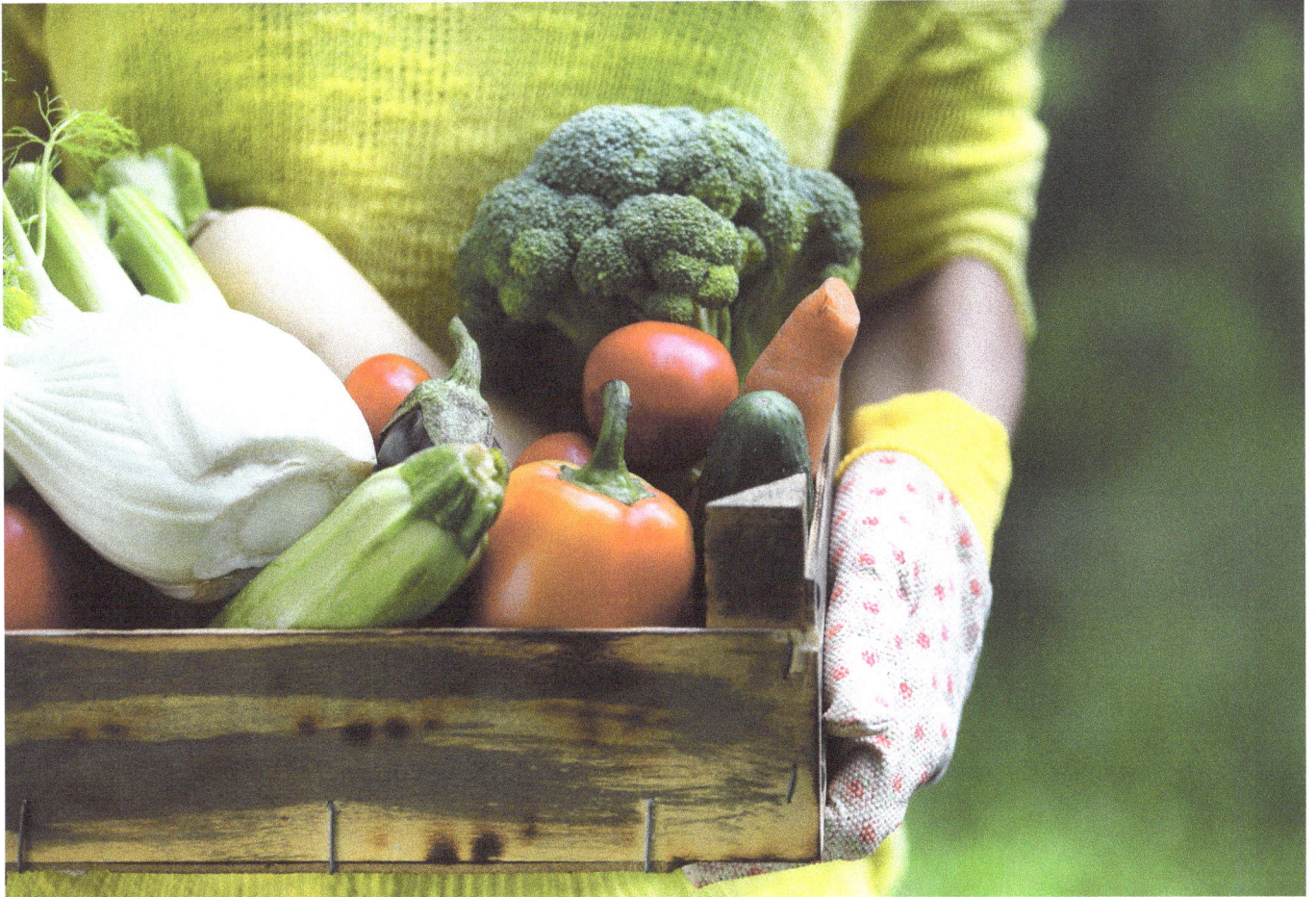

Now that you have completed the 40-Day Wellness Program, do not stop. **Keep living the lifestyle you have just learned, and reap the bountiful benefits and blessings.**

Now it is time to add a 10-Day Prayer Program for the power of the Holy Spirit, just like the disciples did. **PRAY AND WAIT. Each day, pray for the fruits of the Holy Spirit to be reflected in yourself and others.**

Day 1+

Pray for LOVE, which is charity and good will. Pray:

1. to have love for others *(1 Cor. 13)*.
2. to have love for fellow Christians *(1 John 2:10)*.
3. for God's love for us *(John 3:16)*.

Day 2+

Pray for JOY, which is gladness and a rejoicing spirit. Pray:

1. to be filled with joy *(Rom. 15:13)*.
2. for joy in your belief *(1 Peter 1:8)*.

Day 3+

Pray for PEACE, which is harmony, concord, and security. Pray:

1. for the peace of Jesus *(Eph. 2:14)*.
2. for the peace that comes with knowing you are saved in Christ *(Rom. 8:6)*.

Day 4+

Pray for LONGSUFFERING, which is patience, endurance, and steadfastness. Pray:

1. for help in bearing troubles *(Col. 1:11)*.
2. for slowness to avenge wrongs or to become angry *(Rom. 2:4)*.

Day 5+

Pray for GENTLENESS, which is kindness and mercy. Pray:

1. for help in striving for this trait *(Col. 3:12)*.
2. for the same kindness and love for others that God has towards us *(Titus 3:4, 5)*.
3. to perform acts of mercy when needed *(Luke 10:33–35)*.

Day 6+

Pray for GOODNESS, which is uprightness of heart and beneficence. Pray:

1. for a deepening need to be filled with it *(Rom. 15:14)*.
2. for it to be found in you *(Eph. 5:8–9)*.

Day 7+

Pray for FAITH, which is confidence and trust. Pray:

1. to be faithful to Jesus, as He is to us *(Heb. 3:2)*.
2. to be dependable and obedient in all your practices *(Luke 16:10–12)*.

Day 8+

Pray for MEEKNESS, which is to be patient, teachable, and submissive. Pray:

1. to receive omit God's Word with a humble Spirit *(James 1:21)*.
2. for a meek attitude towards all people *(Titus 3:2)*.

Day 9+

Pray for TEMPERANCE, which is self-control and mastering of one's desires. Pray:

1. to overcome weakness so you can continue on the path to godliness *(2 Peter 1:5–7)*.
2. to master anything unhealthful that may be keeping you from a clear mind *(1 Peter 5:8; Isa. 5:22)*.

Day 10+

Pray for **THE HOLY SPIRIT** to help you. Pray:

1. to be holy and acceptable to God *(Rom. 12:1, 2)*.
2. to be a workman that need not to be ashamed *(2 Tim. 3:15)*.

Disclaimer

This journal was created from the author's personal experience, to encourage and guide you through reaching your optimal personal lifestyle. The material is intended for biblical lifestyle education only, and does not take the place of medical advice. You are responsible for any use of the Biblical information mentioned.

For diagnosis of your condition or advice on prescriptions, see your preferred health professional or physician.

For healing, "Behold the LAMB OF GOD, which taketh away the sin of the world" (John 1:20, bold supplied for emphasis). **The Holy Word** says, "And ye shall serve the LORD your God, and he shall bless thy bread, and thy water; and I will take sickness away from the midst of thee" (Ex. 23:25).

He says, *"Behold, I will bring it HEALTH and CURE, and I will cure them, and will reveal unto them the abundance of PEACE and TRUTH"* (Jer. 33:6, capitalization supplied for emphasis).

Appendix: Measurement Conversion Chart

Teaspoon = tsp.

Tablespoon = Tbsp.

Fluid = fl.

Ounce = oz.

Pint = pt.

Quart = qt.

Gallon = gal.

Milliliter = ml.

2 Pinches = ⅛ tsp.

Dash = about ⅛ tsp.

60 drops = 1 tsp. =⅙ fl. oz.

3 tsp. = 1 Tbsp.

1 Tbsp. = 3 tsp. = ½ fl. oz. = 15 ml.

2 Tbsp. = ⅛ cup =1 fl. oz. = 30 ml.

4 Tbsp. = ¼ cup = 2 fl. oz. = 60 ml.

½ cup = 8 Tbsp. = 4 fl. oz. = 120 ml.

1 cup = 16 Tbsp. = 8 fl. oz. = 240 ml. = ½ pt.

2 cups = 16 fl. oz. = 480 ml.= 1 pt.

4 cups = 32 fl. oz. = 2 pt. =1 qt.

8 cups = 64 fl. oz. = 4 pt. = 2 qt.

4 qts. = 1 gal.

¼ tsp. dried herbs = 1 tsp. minced fresh herbs.

Bibliography

Dence, Calvin. Your Heart's Desire, Good Health. The Printers, 1979.

"Facts Statistics: Drowsy Driving." Insurance Information Institute. Insurance Information Institute, Inc. https://1ref.us/19b (accessed Jun. 22, 2020).

Ferrell, Vance, and Harold M. Cherne. Natural Remedies Encyclopedia: Home Remedies for Over 730 Diseases. Altamont, TN: Harvestime Books, 2010.

Foster, Vernon W. M.D. New Start! Weimar, CA: Weimar Institute, 1990.

Hoffmann, Thomas. "Exercise Better for Health than Dietary Changes." ScienceNordic, 11 Apr. 2012. https://1ref.us/19n (accessed Jun. 22, 2020).

Kruse, Kersten. "Behind the Wheel: Reducing Road Rage." A Healthier Michigan, July 23, 2018. https://1ref.us/19c (accessed Jun. 22, 2020).

Kueppers, Pat. "What's More Important: Exercise or Diet?" Allina Health, November 22, 2015. https://1ref.us/19d (accessed Jun. 22, 2020).

Lucas, Frank. "Death Begins in the Colon—Stop It from Happening to You." NUPRO, February 27, 2014. https://1ref.us/19m (accessed Jun. 22, 2020).

McNeilus Mary Ann, M.D. God's Healing Way. Whalan, MN: Mercy Valley Farms, 2010.

Mercola, Joseph. "Top 10 Food Additives to Avoid." Mercola.com, December 17, 2010. https://1ref.us/19e (accessed Jun. 22, 2020).

Ogunjimi, Angela. "Diseases from High Protein Intake." LIVESTRONG.COM. Leaf Group. https://1ref.us/19f (accessed Jun. 22, 2020).

Paulien, Gunther B., Ph.D. The Divine Prescription. Brushton, NY: TEACH Services, Inc., 1997.

Sharma, Sunil, and Mani Kavuru. "Sleep and Metabolism: An Overview." International Journal of Endocrinology 2010 (August 2, 2010): 1–12. https://1ref.us/19g (accessed Jun. 22, 2020).

"Sun Safety." American Skin Association, 2012. https://1ref.us/19h (accessed Jun. 22, 2020).

Thrash, Agatha M. "Clothing: Preventative Medicine." Uchee Pines, September 15, 2013. https://1ref.us/19i (accessed Jun. 22, 2020).

—— "Eating Between Meals: Preventative Medicine." Uchee Pines, September 15, 2013. https://1ref.us/19j (accessed Jun. 22, 2020).

Thrash, Agatha M., Calvin L. Thrash. Home Remedies: Hydrotherapy, Massage, Charcoal and Other Simple Treatments. United States: Thrash Publications, 1981.

Tortora, Gerard J., and Sandra Reynolds. Grabowski. Principles of Anatomy and Physiology. New York: Wiley, 2000.

Vina, J, F Sanchis-Gomar, V Martinez-Bello, and M C Gomez-Cabrera. "Exercise Acts as a Drug; the Pharmacological Benefits of Exercise." British Journal of Pharmacology. Blackwell Publishing Ltd, September 2012. https://1ref.us/19k (accessed Jun. 22, 2020).

Wang, Hao, Chuan-Xian Wei, Lu Min, and Ling-Yun Zhu. "Good or Bad: Gut Bacteria in Human Health and Diseases." Biotechnology & Biotechnological Equipment 32, no. 5 (November 2018): 1075–80. https://1ref.us/19l (accessed Jun. 22, 2020).

White, Ellen G. Counsels on Diet and Foods: A Compilation from the Writings of Ellen G. White. Takoma Park, MD: Review and Herald Pub. Association, 1976.

—— Healthful Living. Brushton, NY: TEACH Services, Inc., 1997.

—— Mind, Character and Personality Vol. 2. Takoma Park, MD: Review and Herald Pub. Association, 2001.

—— Steps to Christ. Mountain View, CA: Pacific Press Publishing Association, 1892.

Zemel, Michael B., Sally A. Schuette, Maren Hegsted, and Hellen M. Linkswiler. "Role of the Sulfur-Containing Amino Acids in Protein-Induced Hypercalciuria in Men." The Journal of Nutrition 111, no. 3 (January 1981): 545–52. https://1ref.us/19o (accessed Jun. 22, 2020).

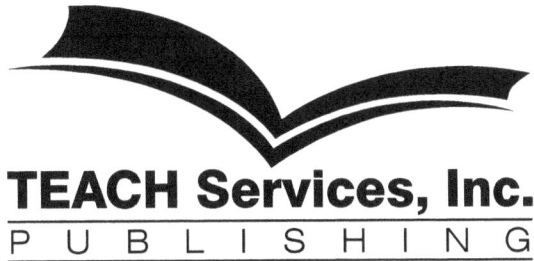

www.ingramcontent.com/pod-product-compliance
Lightning Source LLC
Chambersburg PA
CBHW080242270326
41926CB00020B/4339